Culture, Ethnicity and Chronic C

T0227659

The global burden of chronic non-communicable diseases (NCDs), such as stroke, diabetes and cancers, and of common mental disorders such as depression and anxiety, has a disproportionate impact on the low- and middle-income countries (LMICs) of Africa, Asia and Latin America. The pattern persists in African and Asian migrant populations in European and North American countries, despite the higher standards of living and improved health infrastructure. The consensus of experts is that pragmatic, cost-effective and sustainable interventions are required, and that these must prioritise the social determinants of NCDs as well as the social participation of affected communities. Despite the growing emphasis on the role of social processes in health system responses to chronic disease in LMICs, there has been no definitive volume that brings together LMICs perspectives on these issues.

This book aims to address this major gap by presenting new conceptual and empirical perspectives on the interconnections between culture, ethnicity and chronic conditions in LMICs and their implications for research, intervention and policy. The chapters focus on lay and institutional meanings, experiences and responses to chronic conditions in selected countries in Africa, Europe and the Caribbean.

This book was originally published as a special issue of *Ethnicity and Health*.

Charles Agyemang is Senior Researcher and PI in the Academic Medical Centre, University of Amsterdam, The Netherlands. He is currently the Vice President for the European Public Health Association, Migrant Health section. His research focuses on cardiovascular diseases among ethnic minority and migrant groups in Europe and cardiovascular diseases in LMICs.

Ama de-Graft Aikins is Associate Professor of Social Psychology and Director of the Centre for Social Policy Studies, University of Ghana, and Visiting Senior Fellow at LSE Health, London School of Economics and Political Science. Her research focuses on experiences of, and interventions for, diabetes and related chronic physical and mental conditions.

Culture, Ethnicity and Chronic Conditions

A Global Synthesis

Edited by
Charles Agyemang and Ama de-Graft Aikins

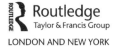
Routledge
Taylor & Francis Group

LONDON AND NEW YORK

First published 2014
by Routledge

Published 2014 by Routledge

2 Park Square, Milton Park, Abingdon, Oxfordshire, OX14 4RN

and by Routledge
711 Third Avenue, New York, NY 10017

Routledge is an imprint of the Taylor and Francis Group, an informa business

First issued in paperback 2015

British Library Cataloguing in Publication Data
A catalogue record for this book is available from the British Library

ISBN 978-0-415-71539-3 (hbk)
ISBN 978-1-138-95396-3 (pbk)

Typeset in Times New Roman
by Taylor & Francis Books

Publisher's Note
The publisher accepts responsibility for any inconsistencies that may have arisen during the conversion of this book from journal articles to book chapters, namely the possible inclusion of journal terminology.

Disclaimer
Every effort has been made to contact copyright holders for their permission to reprint material in this book. The publishers would be grateful to hear from any copyright holder who is not here acknowledged and will undertake to rectify any errors or omissions in future editions of this book.

Contents

CONTENTS

Citation Information

The chapters in this book were originally published in *Ethnicity and Health*, volume 17, issue 6 (December 2012). When citing this material, please use the original page numbering for each article, as follows:

Chapter 1
*Editorial: Culture, ethnicity and chronic conditions: reframing
concepts and methods for research, interventions and policy in low-
and middle-income countries*
Ama de-Graft Aikins, Emma Pitchforth, Pascale Allotey,
Gbenga Ogedegbe and Charles Agyemang
Ethnicity and Health, volume 17, issue 6 (December 2012)
pp. 551–561

Chapter 2
*Editorial: Cardiovascular disease in low- and middle-income countries:
an urgent priority*
Haja R. Wurie and Francesco P. Cappuccio
Ethnicity and Health, volume 17, issue 6 (December 2012)
pp. 543–550

Chapter 3
*Ethnicity and cardiovascular health research: pushing the boundaries
by including comparison populations in the countries of origin*
Charles Agyemang, Ama de-Graft Aikins and Raj Bhopal
Ethnicity and Health, volume 17, issue 6 (December 2012)
pp. 579–596

Chapter 4
*'A chronic disease is a disease which keeps coming back . . . it is like
the flu': chronic disease risk perception and explanatory models among French-
and Swahili-speaking African migrants*
Maxwell Cooper, Seeromanie Harding, Kenneth Mullen and
Catherine O'Donnell
Ethnicity and Health, volume 17, issue 6 (December 2012)
pp. 597–613

Chapter 5
*Explanatory models of hypertension among Nigerian patients at
a University Teaching Hospital*
Kelly D. Taylor, Ayoade Adedokun, Olugbenga Awobusuyi,
Peju Adeniran, Elochukwu Onyia and Gbenga Ogedegbe
Ethnicity and Health, volume 17, issue 6 (December 2012)
pp. 615–629

Chapter 6
*Coping and chronic psychosocial consequences of female genital
mutilation in the Netherlands*
Erick Vloeberghs, Anke van der Kwaak, Jeroen Knipscheer and
Maria van den Muijsenbergh
Ethnicity and Health, volume 17, issue 6 (December 2012)
pp. 677–695

Chapter 7
*Differences in working conditions and employment arrangements
among migrant and non-migrant workers in Europe*
Elena Ronda Pérez, Fernando G. Benavides, Katia Levecque,
John G. Love, Emily Felt and Ronan Van Rossem
Ethnicity and Health, volume 17, issue 6 (December 2012)
pp. 563–577

Chapter 8
*Review of community-based interventions for prevention of cardiovascular
diseases in low- and middle-income countries*
Steven van de Vijver, Samuel Oti, Juliet Addo, Ama de-Graft Aikins and
Charles Agyemang
Ethnicity and Health, volume 17, issue 6 (December 2012)
pp. 651–676

Chapter 9
*Policy initiatives, culture and the prevention and control of chronic
non-communicable diseases (NCDs) in the Caribbean*
T. Alafia Samuels, Cornelia Guell, Branka Legetic and Nigel Unwin
Ethnicity and Health, volume 17, issue 6 (December 2012)
pp. 631–649

Please direct any queries you may have about the citations to
clsuk.permissions@cengage.com

INTRODUCTION

Culture, ethnicity and chronic conditions: reframing concepts and methods for research, interventions and policy in low- and middle-income countries

Chronic physical and mental conditions constitute a significant proportion of the global burden of disease. Low- and middle-income countries (LMICs) of Africa, Asia, Latin America and the Caribbean are disproportionately affected. According to the World Health Organization (WHO) (2008), four major chronic non-communicable diseases (NCDs) – cardiovascular diseases (CVD), cancers, chronic respiratory diseases and diabetes – cause an estimated 60% of all global deaths, with an estimated 80% of these deaths occurring in LMICs. Similarly, an estimated 14% of the global disease burden is attributable to common mental disorders like depression and anxiety disorders; almost 75% of these disorders occur in LMICs (WHO 2010). In high-income countries of Europe and North America, the pattern of high chronic disease risk, disability and death persists among migrant populations from Africa, Asia and the Caribbean, despite higher standards of living and improved health infrastructure (Agyemang et al. 2009; Davies et al. 2011; Dressler et al. 2005).

The burden of chronic diseases in LMICs has been attributed to an interaction of factors including rapid urbanisation, ageing populations, globalisation, poor lifestyle practices and poverty (Beaglehole et al. 2011). While these factors are recognised, the development of solutions presents complex challenges because LMIC health systems struggle to address a cumulative burden of infectious and chronic diseases, and chronic disease research, intervention and policies are limited. For migrant populations in Europe and North America, the complexities arise from the diverse structures of immigration policies and the politics of minority ethnic inclusion in social, political and health systems (Agyemang et al. 2009; Dressler et al. 2005; Oppenheimer 2001; Phinney et al. 2001). The consensus of experts, endorsed by the UN High level meeting on NCDs in September 2011, is that given the health systems deficiencies in chronic disease care in LMICs, pragmatic, cost-effective and sustainable interventions are required and these must prioritise the social determinants of NCDs as well as the social participation of affected communities (Beaglehole et al. 2011; de-Graft Aikins et al. 2010a; United Nations 2011; Marmot 2005).

Despite the growing emphasis on the role of social processes in health systems responses to chronic disease in LMICs there has been no definitive volume that brings together LMIC perspectives on these issues. Influential international journals – for example, *Lancet, WHO Bulletin, International Journal of Epidemiology, International Health, International Journal for Equity in Health, Plos Medicine, Globalization and Health, Tropical Medicine & International Health* – have published review papers on NCDs in LMICs. These reviews have focused on the epidemiological and health

1

systems aspects of the burden. Existing books that tackle the burden of NCDs with reference to LMICs have either focused on a structural aspect of the NCD burden, for example, economic (Suhrcke et al. 2006) and public policy (Adeyi, Smith, and Robles 2007), or on single conditions, for example, CVD (Labarthe 2010) and child obesity (Waters et al. 2010). No definitive text or volume exists that synthesises the complex multi-level dimensions of chronic physical and mental conditions in LMICs from the perspective of sociocultural processes and responses.

This *Ethnicity and Health* special issue, titled *Culture, Ethnicity and Chronic Condition: a Global Synthesis*, aims to address this key gap by presenting new conceptual and empirical perspectives on the interconnections between culture, ethnicity and chronic conditions in LMICs and their implications for research, intervention and policy. The articles focus on lay and institutional meanings, experiences and responses to chronic conditions in selected countries in Africa, Europe and the Caribbean. The idea for the issue developed from an international symposium, *Prioritising Chronicity: an agenda for public health research on chronic disease for sub-Saharan Africa and Asia*, held in Kuala Lumpur, Malaysia in 2010. Convened by Monash University, Malaysia and the British Academy funded UK–Africa Academic Partnership on Chronic Disease, the aim of the symposium was to examine the impact of chronic conditions on health systems in LMICs and to explore the potential for cross-fertilization of African and Asian research, intervention and policy. Some articles in this issue were either initially presented at the symposium or developed by symposium participants specifically for this call.

The chronic conditions and communities in focus

The chronic conditions in focus fall under two categories: (1) chronic physical conditions and their risk factors (Agyemang et al. forthcoming; Cooper et al. 2012; Samuels et al. 2012; Taylor et al. forthcoming; van de Vijver et al. 2013); and (2) chronic mental health and psychosocial conditions and their social determinants (Ronda et al. forthcoming; Vloeberghs et al. forthcoming). The research communities described in the empirical papers include Nigerians of mixed ethnicities (Yoruba, Ibo, other) living with hypertension in Lagos, Nigeria (Taylor et al. forthcoming), African migrants of mixed nationalities (Burundi, Democratic Republic of Congo, Republic of Congo, Rwanda, Somalia, Tanzania, Uganda) living in Glasgow making sense of chronic diseases and their risk factors (Cooper et al. 2012), migrant African women of mixed nationalities (Eritrea, Ethiopia, Sierra Leone, Somalia, Sudan) living in the Netherlands recounting their home country experiences of female genital mutilation or cutting (FGM/C; Vloeberghs et al. forthcoming), and migrants of various nationalities self-reporting their health disabling working conditions through the European Working Conditions Survey conducted in all 31 European countries (Ronda et al. forthcoming). The conceptual articles examine structural responses to NCDs in the Caribbean region (Samuels et al. 2012) and to CVD in LMICs (van de Vijver et al. 2013) and among African, African-Caribbean and Asian migrant communities in Europe and North America (Agyemang et al. forthcoming). All three articles place emphasis on the interacting, and mutually reinforcing, roles of national policies, health systems processes and research cultures in structural responses to NCDs in these diverse contexts.

The articles demonstrate the importance of culture, ethnicity and broader social conditions in multi-level responses to chronic conditions. They also point to the need for reframing these concepts in order to develop more robust research, interventions and policies in LMICs and for LMIC migrants living in high-income European countries. We focus on these emerging conceptual themes in the sections that follow.

Culture and chronic conditions: a multi-level, polyphasic and dynamic approach

Samuels et al. (2012) provide a useful set of definitions of culture which operates at different levels of social organisation. Citing Eckersley (2007, 194), Samuels et al. (2012) define culture as 'the language and accumulated knowledge, beliefs, practices, assumptions and values that are passed between individuals, groups and generations'. This common definition of culture fixes attention to the culture of lay societies. Samuels et al. (2012) also define culture as a 'complex and multifaceted' concept that is variably distributed between generations and populations and is influenced by local, political and economic factors. This definition underscores culture in its 'widest possible remit' by taking on the macro-structure elements of society, including the culture of formal institutions, nations and geopolitical systems. This multi-level concept of culture is evident in a number of articles in this special issue.

At a fundamental level, the culture(s) of lay societies informs individual health and illness beliefs, knowledge, experiences and actions. Taylor et al. (forthcoming) report that explanatory models of hypertension among Nigerians with hypertension draw on traditional health beliefs of physical disorder, common sense observations of the relationship between life stressors and ill health, biomedical models of hypertension provided by health professionals and religious models of coping and spiritually mediated cures. Cooper et al. (2012) report that Eastern and Central African migrants in Glasgow make sense of chronic diseases through the lens of dominant representations of diseases in their home countries, individual and family health status, biomedical knowledge gained from doctors and their everyday perceptions of existing diseases in Glasgow. Migrant African women in the Netherlands who have experienced FGM/C make sense of their experiences through the lens of their cultural traditions, religion, family support systems, social and advocacy networks and the Dutch health system (Vloeberghs et al. forthcoming).

In the Nigerian and Scottish research settings the lay knowledge of chronic diseases presented is not completely aligned with ideal biomedical models; the misalignment has health implications. In the Nigerian setting misconceptions about the causes and prognosis for hypertension are likely to undermine appropriate self-management of hypertension. In the Glasgow setting low awareness of chronic disease risk, based on false dichotomies constructed between a higher risk of infectious diseases among Africans and higher risk of chronic diseases among Europeans, is likely to undermine the adoption of healthy lifestyles by African migrants. In the Netherlands, a combination of the psychosocial and stigmatising impact of FGM/C and barriers to culturally appropriate care in the Dutch health system place some women in positions of isolation and silent suffering. In all three studies, these problems do not rise solely from the use of traditional cultural knowledge and beliefs. Study participants draw, consciously and eclectically, from different systems of knowledge, including their indigenous traditions, to make sense of the chronic conditions under study. This cognitive process is theoretically significant.

'Cognitive polyphasia' is a social psychological concept of social knowledge production that suggests that in everyday life, across a variety of cultures, individuals and communities draw on diverse, and even opposing, models of knowledge (Moscovici 2008; Provencher 2011). Syntheses of qualitative research on everyday responses to diabetes and hypertension experiences suggest that cognitive polyphasia may be a universal response to the complex – biological, psychological, sociocultural and material – impact of living with a long-term chronic condition (Campbell et al. 2003; Marshall, Wolfe, and McKevitt 2012). Depending on the context and personal goals, this process of knowledge production may be psychologically difficult or easy for the individual. Taylor et al. (forthcoming), for example, interpret the psychological impact of contradictory hypertension knowledge among their Nigerian participants in terms of 'cognitive dissonance' (Festinger 1957), the psychological tension, or discomfort that arises from holding inconsistent beliefs or expressing inconsistent behaviours. Psychological ease or comfort with inconsistent thinking and behaviour – the opposite of cognitive dissonance – is also possible and more common than reported and theorised (Markova 2003; de-Graft Aikins 2012). A systematic review of qualitative research on lay perspectives on hypertension and drug adherence in 16 countries across six regions (Africa, Asia, Australia, Europe, North America and South America) conducted by Marshall, Wolfe, and McKevitt (2012) suggested remarkable similarities in lay knowledge of the causes and consequences of hypertension. The sources of knowledge were eclectic and 'individual participants often held mutually contradictory explanations, and the inconsistencies did not trouble them'. There is a tendency within global public health to view health and illness beliefs in the western context (usually denoting high-income countries of Europe and North America) as rational and health and illness beliefs in non-western cultures (most LMICs) as faulty and irrational, particularly among the uneducated rural poor. This perception influences the development of education and related interventions. The review of community-based interventions for the prevention of CVDs in LMICs, conducted by Van der Vijver et al. (2013) underscores the limitations of adopting such dichotomies. The review suggests that public health education provided via the mass media, in workplaces, schools and in communities is more successful in changing some health behaviours when combined with improving primary healthcare, including access to affordable medicines. However, positive behaviour change appears to be influenced by personal proximity to or experience of CVD and may fluctuate over time, especially in the absence of follow-up care and intervention monitoring. This evidence is similar to evidence gathered in high-income countries on the limitations of KAB (knowledge–attitude–behaviour) approaches to health behaviour change and of cross-sectional interventions for chronic illness management (Crossley 2000; Campbell et al. 2003; Joffe 2002). KAB critics argue, and have demonstrated, that the relationship between knowledge, attitudes and behaviour is not linear or predictable, because this relationship is mediated by the complex dynamics of social life, relationships, resources and goals. Similarly, the healthcare and self-care strategies of the chronically ill are not linear or predictable because the experience of chronic disease is lifelong and unfolds within the complex dynamics of biological, psychological, social and material changes. These emerging perspectives on the complex use of knowledge for rational purposes across cultural contexts suggest there is a need for a change in conceptual approaches to public health education and healthcare. First, interventions should recognise, legitimise and incorporate lay perspectives or explanatory models (Taylor et al. forthcoming; Cooper et al. 2012). Second, the success of interventions will depend on the extent to which the psychological functions – positive, negative, benign – of eclectic knowledge production are understood. Finally, longitudinal approaches are required to understand and address the impact of time and chronicity on healthcare and self-care strategies. Methods that capture depth and complexity of knowledge, experiences and social practices, such as the qualitative approaches described in this issue, will be most appropriate to these research issues.

The role of culture at the level of macro-structures is evident in the structural context and structural responses to the rising prevalence of NCDs in the Caribbean (Samuels et al. 2012). It is also salient in the diversity of working conditions of migrant populations across Europe (Ronda et al. forthcoming) and the ideological framework of research on ethnic minority health in Europe and North America (Agyemang et al. forthcoming). Samuels et al. (2012) present a nuanced account of the way the social determinants of NCD risk and morbidity in the Caribbean are shaped by current poverty and social inequalities in countries like Haiti, as well as by a shared history of slavery and the effects of slavery on family systems, gender relations and gendered and class-based health practices across much of the region. They demonstrate the way these historical and economic forces have also shaped the culture of governance and policy-making particularly in the areas of social development, the development of strategic regional partnerships and the adoption of global policies. The national or regional adoption of NCD policies have to be understood within this context.

In their analysis of the impact of working conditions on the physical and psychosocial health of migrants, Ronda et al. (forthcoming) observe 'different [European] countries with distinct cultures, attitudes and regulations' engender different 'working conditions and employment arrangements'. This idea of the interaction between national 'cultures, attitudes and regulations' and lay cultures attitudes and everyday practices cuts across the discussions on structural responses to chronic diseases and psychosocial problems in the European and Caribbean regions. Within this interpretive framework, the transformation of research, intervention and policy in LMICs and in high-income countries with migrant populations from LMICs rests on two requirements. First, expert and policy cultures have to be open to, and collaborate with, lay communities, in terms of incorporating lay knowledge, everyday practices and agency into the development of interventions. Second, expert and policy communities have to learn from best practices and relevant policies across national and regional borders. The ideas expressed here are strongly aligned with ecological and multi-level models of public health and health policy, which suggest mutual inter-relationships between individual, social, environmental and structural dimensions (Hepworth 2004; Richard et al. 2011; Whitehead 2007). A key, and crucial difference, is that they explicitly introduce a fifth layer of geopolitical engagement and participation within this model.

Ethnicity and chronic conditions: addressing complexity and dynamism of communities

Ethnicity, ethnic groups, ethnic minority groups and migrant groups are used interchangeably to describe research communities in this issue. Agyemang et al. (forthcoming) define ethnicity as 'the group a person belongs to as a result of a mix of cultural factors including language, diet, religion and ancestry' and ethnic minority group, in the European context, as 'minority populations of non European origin'. Ethnicity is a useful concept for public health research because, as a social construct, it facilitates the examination of attitudes, beliefs and practices relevant to a delineated group (Oppenheimer 2001). However, ethnicity is also a problematic concept because, as Agyemang et al. (forthcoming) point out, there are no appropriate terms for its use in the scientific study of health. On the one hand, the constituents of ethnicity presented in the first definition – shared language, diet, religion and ancestry – are very similar to the constituents of culture. At a conceptual and methodological level it raises questions about where culture ends and ethnicity begins in contexts of social diversity. On the other hand, the use of ethnicity within the context of 'ethnic minority' discourse in Europe and North America tends to obscure national differences (e.g. Nigerian versus Ghanaian, Jamaican versus Trinidadian and Indian versus Bangladeshi) and ethnic differences within different nationalities (e.g. Yoruba versus Ibo within the Nigerian nationality). Cultural and social theorists have argued that references to 'minority ethnic' status capture 'politics of recognition' rather than the psychology of agentic identity construction and use (Knowles 2010). As Oppenheimer (2001, 1053) observes ethnic group 'is often used to connote a people outside of, alien to, and different from the core population' and is 'associated with relatively recent immigration, with discrimination and prejudice or the perception of being marginally White or non-White, with the need to overcome marginal economic, political and social status'.

This ideological position is limited and tends to ignore the growing evidence on the agency of minority ethnic groups in local and global socio-political spheres, for example, through political participation and cultural advocacy in their host and home countries (Bagwell 2008; Jaegers 2008) and economic support of their home countries through remittances (Page and Plaza 2006). Furthermore, focusing on minority ethnic groups through the lens of political identity obscures the importance and nuances of self-identification.

Social psychological, sociological and cultural theories of social identity, ethnicity and multiculturalism suggest that the process of self-identification is complex (Elwert 1995; Knowles 2010; Phinney et al. 2001). Elwert's (1995) concept of polytaxis – defined as a 'latent multiplicity of order' – underscores the idea that in everyday interactions and practices, individuals draw on and use multiple identities based on their membership to diverse social groups and on their particular needs in specific social situations. Ethnicity, in this formulation, constitutes one of several functional legitimate identities. As Cooper et al. (2012) observe that there is great diversity in dietary practices, culture, language use, religious faith and personal migration history that impinge on perceptions of health and well-being and on chronic disease risk among African migrants. Indeed, this interplay of diversity and complexity is manifested in the way coping strategies and styles of migrant African women who have undergone FGM/C differ depending on nationality, age, educational status, quality of family support and access to broader social and religious support systems (Vloeberghs et al. forthcoming).

Epidemiological and public health research may use broad, externally imposed, categories of nationality, ethnicity and migrant status to illuminate important demographic differences of risk, morbidity and mortality within and across countries (Agyemang et al. 2005; Oppenheimer 2001). However, at the level of interventions in concrete social settings, it is important that approaches focus on the nuances between, across and beyond these categories.

Agyemang et al. (forthcoming) synthesise evidence on the cardiovascular health status of African, African-Caribbean and Asian migrants in Europe and North America. They show that these migrant populations, in general, have poorer health outcomes compared to the majority populations in their host countries. Some groups from West Africa, Asia and South East Asia are reported to have poorer cardiovascular health status compared to their compatriots in their home countries. This evidence has complex roots and consequences. First, the local situation of ethnic minority and migrant populations may vary greatly across nations and these national contextual differences can influence the health of these populations in different ways. Second, the health status of the local reference host population will ultimately determine the relative health standing of the ethnic minority and migrant groups within the country in which they live. They refer to this phenomenon as 'migrant pond effect' or 'migrant context effect'. Agyemang et al. (forthcoming) observe that the dominant focus of research has been on researching ethnic or migrant groups in their host countries. This has obscured nuances between biological, social and structural factors in risk, morbidity and mortality. They argue that future research will be enriched by extending ethnicity and health research across national borders, by either comparing similar ethnic or migrant groups living in different locations within a region, or comparing ethnic or migrant populations with similar populations in their country of origin. They describe a multi-site research project on Ghanaians living in three European countries (Germany, the Netherlands and the UK) and in rural and urban Ghana that is likely to offer insights on the complex inter-relationship between ethnicity and health across the migration divide.

The implications for research are fourfold. First, as Oppenheimer (2001) suggests, and several authors do in this issue, researchers must define their construction of ethnicity (or related concept) and justify its validity, reliability and consistency for their studies. Second, researchers have to be conceptually and methodologically sensitive to the mutual constitution of the subjective, social and material dimensions of ethnicity (Gunaratnam 2003; Dressler et al. 2005). Third, the limits of ethnicity must be recognised, in cases where individuals and groups apply alternative social categories to make sense of themselves, their understandings of health and diseases and of their positions in relation to health and disease. Finally, investment in multi-site studies that hold ethnicity and related social categories constant will bring these complex dynamics to the fore.

Conclusions

NCDs have typically been perceived as conditions of wealth and ageing. By extension they have been perceived as problems of high-income countries with large ageing populations. Current evidence suggests that this is a misconception. LMICs are now experiencing a higher NCD burden and this is occurring across regions regardless of the wealth status of countries or the dynamics of ageing. In fact, in LMICs, NCD morbidity and mortality appears to occur at younger ages and poor communities are disproportionately affected. Frenk et al. (1989) have attributed these processes to a 'protracted polarised' model of the epidemiological transition. The model suggests that in LMICs a protracted double burden of infectious and chronic diseases has existed over time. Second, the burden of chronic diseases is polarised across socio-economic status, with wealthy communities experiencing high chronic disease risk and poor communities experiences a double burden of infectious and chronic diseases. A major challenge in the future, as Van der Vijver et al. (2013) observe, will be the development of chronic disease interventions for growing urban slum populations in LMICs.

Health systems in LMICs are weak and there are challenges in health care provisions for migrants from LMICs in high-income countries. Political, economic and policy factors play a major role in this cross-cutting problem. But the problem lies also in limited research approaches of describing affected communities, understanding their circumstances and capturing the nuances of their perspectives on the causes and consequences of chronic conditions.

As the empirical articles in this issue have shown, sociocultural systems and processes mediate community and individual responses to chronic disease risk, experiences and healthcare, and often in unpredictable ways. Health and illness beliefs and practices rooted in cultural systems, complementary and alternative medical systems operating outside formal biomedical institutions, and everyday health information and advice from family, friends, workplace, advocacy organisations and the mass media present legitimate, but also contentious, sources for making sense of the scale, proximity and impact of chronic diseases in the public sphere (see also BeLue et al. 2009; de-Graft Aikins et al. 2010b; Marshall, Wolfe, and McKevitt 2012; Setel 2003; Whyte 2012). Individuals and groups draw on different, often contradictory, systems of knowledge to make sense of illness and develop evolving strategies for illness experiences.

Social identity, like social knowledge, is complex and can be put to diverse uses by individuals, communities and institutions. Individuals may draw on diverse social identities in their everyday life, depending on their membership to groups structured along cultural, ethnic, gendered, socio-economic and other socially relevant lines. Ethnicity is an important social construct in public health and epidemiological research on migrant populations in high-income countries and in LMICs. However, its use has not reflected the complexity of functional social identities in the lives of research communities. We have discussed how the articles in this issue provide insights for reframing ethnicity for more robust research. To operationalize culture and ethnicity in a meaningful way, conceptual and methodological frameworks have to be multi-level (by focusing on the mutual inter-relationship between the individual, social, environmental, structural and geopolitical), polyphasic (by recognising the latent multiplicity of knowledge and identities) and dynamic (by paying attention to time and chronicity). Investment in multi-site, multidisciplinary and mixed methods studies will illuminate these nuances in concrete ways to aid pragmatic and sustainable interventions targeted at mitigating the rising epidemic of NCDs in LMICs.

Ama de-Graft Aikins[a,b], Emma Pitchforth[b,c], Pascale Allotey[d], Gbenga Ogedegbe[e] and Charles Agyemang[f]

[a]Regional Institute for Population Studies, University of Ghana, Accra, Ghana; [b]LSE Health, London School of Economics and Political Science, London WC2 2AE, UK; [c]RAND Europe, Cambridge, UK; [d]School of Medicine and Health Sciences, Monash University, Malaysia; [e]Department of Population Health, Division of Health and

Behavior, New York University School of Medicine, NY, USA; [f]Department of Public Health, Academic Medical Centre, University of Amsterdam, Amsterdam, The Netherlands

References

Adeyi, O., O. Smith, S. Robles. 2007. *Public Policy and the Challenge of Chronic Noncommunicable Diseases (Directions in Development Series)*. Washington, DC: World Bank Publications.

Agyemang, C., R. Bhopal, and M. Bruijnzeels. 2005. "Negro, Black, Black African, African Caribbean, African American or What? Labelling African Origin Populations in the Health Arena in the 21st Century." *Journal of Epidemiology & Community Health* 59 (12): 1014–1018. doi:10.1136/jech.2005.035964.

Agyemang, C., J. Addo, R. Bhopal, A. de Graft Aikins, and K. Stronks. 2009. "Cardiovascular Disease, Diabetes and Established Risk Factors among Populations of Sub-Saharan African Descent in Europe: A Literature Review." *Globalization and Health* 5 (1): 7. doi:10.1186/1744-8603-5-7.

Agyemang, C., A. de-Graft Aikins, and R. Bhopal. Forthcoming. "Ethnicity and Cardiovascular Health Research: Pushing the Boundaries by Including Comparison Populations in the Countries of Origin", *Ethnicity and Health*.

Bagwell, S. 2008. "Transnational Family Networks and Ethnic Minority Business Development. The Case of Vietnamese Nail-shops in the UK." *International Journal of Entrepreneurial Behaviour & Research* 14 (6): 377–394. doi:10.1108/13552550810910960.

Beaglehole, R., R. Bonita, G. Alleyne, R. Horton, L. Li, P. Lincoln, J. C. Mbanya, et al. 2011. "UN High-Level Meeting on Non-Communicable Diseases: Addressing four Questions." *Lancet* 378 (9789): 449–455. doi:10.1016/S0140-6736(11)60879-9.

BeLue, R., T.A. Okoror, J. Iwelunmor, K. D. Taylor, A. N. Degboe, C. Agyemang, and O. Ogedegbe. 2009. "An Overview of Cardiovascular Risk Factor Burden in Sub-Saharan African Countries: A Socio-Cultural Perspective." *Globalization and Health* 5: 10. doi:10.1186/1744-8603-5-10.

Campbell, R., P. Pound, C. Pope, N. Britten, R. Pill, M. Morgan, and J. Donovan. 2003. "Evaluating Meta-Ethnography: A Synthesis of Qualitative Research on Lay Experiences of Diabetes and Diabetes Care." *Social Science & Medicine* 56 (4): 671–684. doi:10.1016/S0277-9536(02)00064-3.

Cooper, M., S. Harding, K. Mullen, and C. O'Donnell. 2012. "A Chronic Disease is a Disease which Keeps Coming Back...it is like the flu": Chronic Disease Risk Perception and Explanatory Models among French and Swahili Speaking African Migrants", *Ethnicity and Health*. doi:10.1080/13557858.2012.740003.

Crossley, M. 2000. *Rethinking Health Psychology*. Buckingham: Open University Press.

Davies, A. A., C. Blake, and P. Dhavan. 2011. "Social Determinants and Risk Factors for Non-Communicable Diseases (NCDs) in South Asian Migrant Populations in Europe." *Asia Europe Journal* 8 (4): 461–473. doi:10.1007/s10308-011-0291-1.

de-Graft Aikins, A. 2012. "Familiarising the Unfamiliar: Cognitive Polyphasia, Emotions and the Creation of Social Representations." *Papers on Social Representations* 21: 7.1–7.28. http://www.psych.lse.ac.uk/psr/.

de-Graft Aikins, A., P. Boynton, and L. L. Atanga. 2010b "Developing Effective Chronic Disease Interventions in Africa: Insights from Ghana and Cameroon." *Globalization and Health* 6: 6. doi:10.1186/1744-8603-6-6

de-Graft Aikins, A., N. Unwin, C. Agyemang, P. Allotey, C. Campbell, and D. K. Arhinful. 2010a. "Tackling Africa's Chronic Disease Burden: From the Local to the Global." *Globalization and Health* 6: 5. doi:10.1186/1744-8603-6-5.

Dressler, W. W., K. S. Oths, and C. C. Gravlee. 2005. "Race and Ethnicity in Public Health Research: Models to Explain Health Disparities." *Annual Review of Anthropology* 34: 231–252. doi:10.1146/annurev.anthro.34.081804.120505.

Eckersley, R. M. 2007. "Culture." In *Macrosocial Determinants of Population Health*, edited by S. Galea, 193–209. New York: Springer.

Elwert, G. 1995. "Boundaries, Cohesion and Switching. On We-Groups in Ethnic, National and Religious Forms." *Bulletin de l'APAD*, 10. http://apad.revues.org/1111 (accessed June 27 2012).

Festinger, L. A. 1957. *A Theory of Cognitive Dissonance*. Stanford: Stanford University Press.

Frenk, J., J. L. Bobadilla, J. Sepulveda, and M. L. Cervantes. 1989. "Health Transition in Middle-income Countries: New Challenges for Health Care." *Health Policy and Planning* 4 (1): 29–39. doi:10.1093/heapol/4.1.29.

Gunaratnam, Y. 2003. *Researching Race and Ethnicity: Methods, Knowledge and Power*. London: Sage.

Hepworth, J. 2004. "Public Health Psychology: A Conceptual and Practical Framework." *Journal of Health Psychology* 9: 41–54. doi:10.1177/1359105304036101.

Jaegers, T. 2008. "Supporting Entrepreneurial Diversity in Europe – Ethnic Minority Entrepreneurship/Migrant Entrepreneurship." *Migrações Journal* 3: 281–284. http://www.oi.acidi.gov.pt/docs/Revista_3_EN/Migr3_Sec4_Art1_EN.pdf.

Joffe, H. 2002. "Social Representations and Health Psychology." *Social Science Information* 41 (4): 559–580. doi:10.1177/0539018402041004004.

Knowles, C. 2010. "Theorizing Race and Ethnicity: Contemporary Paradigms and Perspectives." In *The SAGE Handbook of Race and Ethnic Studies*, edited by P. Hill Collins and J Solomons. London: Sage Publications.

Labarthe, D. R. 2010. *Epidemiology and Prevention of Cardiovascular Disease: A Global Challenge*. Sudbury, MA: Jones & Bartlett Publishers.

Markova, I. 2003. *Dialogicality and Social Representations. The Dynamics of Mind*. Cambridge: Cambridge University Press.

Marmot, M. 2005. "Social Determinants of Health Inequalities." *Lancet* 365: 1099–1104. doi:10.1016/S0140-6736(05)71146-6.

Marshall, I. J., C. D. A. Wolfe, and C. McKevitt. 2012. "Lay Perspectives on Hypertension and Drug Adherence: Systematic Review of Qualitative Research." *BMJ* 344: e3953. doi:10.1136/bmj.e3953.

Moscovici, S. 2008. *Psychoanalysis. Its Image and Its Public*. Cambridge: Polity Press.

Oppenheimer, G. M. 2001. "Paradigm Lost: Race, Ethnicity, and the Search for a New Population Taxonomy." *American Journal of Public Health* 91 (7): 1049–1055. doi:10.2105/AJPH.91.7.1049.

Page, J., and S. Plaza. 2006. "Migration Remittances and Development: A Review of Global Evidence." *Journal of African Economies* 00 (AERC Suppl. 2): 245–336. doi:10.1093/jae/ejl035.

Phinney, J. S., G. Horenczyk, K. Liebkind, and P. Vedder. 2001. "Ethnic Identity, Immigration, and Well-Being: An Interactional Perspective." *Journal of Social Issues* 56 (3): 493–510. doi:10.1111/0022-4537.00225.

Provencher, C. 2011. "Towards a Better Understanding of Cognitive Polyphasia." *Journal for the Theory of Social Behaviour* 41 (4): 377–395. doi:10.1111/j.1468-5914.2011.00468.x.

Richard, L., L. Gauvin, and K. Raine. 2011. "Ecological Models Revisited: Their Uses and Evolution in Health Promotion Over Two Decades." *Annual Review of Public Health* 32 (1): 307–326. doi:10.1146/annurev-publhealth-031210-101141.

Ronda, E., F. G. Benavides, K. Levecque, J. Love, E. Felt, and R. Van Rossem. Forthcoming. "Differences in Working Conditions and Employment Arrangements among Migrant and Non-migrant Workers in Europe", *Ethnicity and Health*.

Samuels, T. A., C. Guell, B. Legetic, and N. Unwin. 2012. "Policy Initiatives, Culture and the Prevention and Control of Chronic Non-Communicable Disease (NCDs) in the Caribbean", *Ethnicity and Health*. doi:10.1080/13557858.2012.752072.

Setel, P. W. 2003. "Non-Communicable Diseases, Political Economy, and Culture in Africa: Anthropological Applications in an Emerging Pandemic." *Ethnicity and Disease* 13 (2 Suppl. 2): S149–S157. http://www.ishib.org/wordpress/?page_id=535.

Suhrcke, M., R. A. Nugent, D. Stuckler, and L. Rocco. 2006. *Chronic Disease: An Economic Perspective*. London: Oxford Health Alliance.

Taylor, K. D., A. Adedokun, O. Awobusuyi, P. Adeniran, E. Onyia, and G. Ogedegbe. Forthcoming. "Explanatory Models of Hypertension among Nigerian Patients at a University Teaching Hospital", *Ethnicity and Health*.

United Nations. 2011. "Draft Political Declaration of the High-level Meeting on the Prevention and Control of Non-Communicable Diseases." September 2011. http://www.un.org/en/ga/ncdmeeting2011/pdf/NCD_draft_political_declaration.pdf (accessed February 21 2012).

van der Vijver, S., S. Oti, J. Addo, A. de-Graft Aikins, and C. Agyemang. 2013. "Systematic Review of Community Based Interventions for Prevention of Cardiovascular Diseases in Low- and Middle-Income Countries", *Ethnicity and Health*. doi:10.1080/13557858.2012.754409.

Vloeberghs, E., A. van der Kwaak, J. Knipscheer, and M. van den Muijsenbergh. Forthcoming. "Coping and Chronic Psychosocial Consequences of Female Genital Mutilation in the Netherlands", *Ethnicity and Health*.

Waters, E., B. Swinburn, J. Seidell, and R. Uauy, eds., 2010. *Preventing Childhood Obesity: Evidence Policy and Practice*. West Sussex: Wiley-Blackwell

Whitehead, M. 2007. "A Typology of Actions to Tackle Social Inequalities in Health." *Journal of Epidemiology and Community Health* 61: 473–478. doi:10.1136/jech.2005.037242.

Whyte, S. R. 2012. "Chronicity and Control: Framing 'noncommunicable diseases' in Africa." *Anthropology & Medicine* 19 (1): 63–74. doi:10.1080/13648470.2012.660465.

World Health Organization WHO. 2008. *2008–2013 Action Plan for the Global Strategy for the Prevention and Control of Noncommunicable Diseases: Prevent and Control Cardiovascular Diseases, Cancers, Chronic Respiratory Diseases and Diabetes*. Geneva: WHO.

WHO. 2010. *mhGAP Intervention Guide for Mental, Neurological and Substance Use Disorders in Non-Specialized Settings*. Geneva: WHO.

Cardiovascular disease in low- and middle-income countries: an urgent priority

Cardiovascular disease burden in low- and middle-income countries (LMICs)

Cardiovascular disease (CVD) is a major global public health crisis, being responsible for 30% of worldwide deaths in 2008 (17 million deaths worldwide from an annual total of 57 million deaths) with an alarming 80% of these deaths occurring in LMICs (WHO 2011). Whilst effective measures are being put in place in high-income countries resulting in a decline in the rate of CVD (Ebrahim et al. 2013), CVD mortality is on a steady rise in LMICs with rates of up to 300–600 deaths attributed to CVD per 100,000 population, and is projected to increase causing preventable loss of lives (WHO 2011). This upsurge of the CVD epidemic poses an additional burden on the already over-burdened health care systems in these settings creating critical challenges to both national health systems and policy development which can impede the development of a strategic plan to address the CVD epidemic. The uncontrolled CVD epidemic is associated with increasing socio-economic costs with high levels of disability and loss of productivity, exacerbating poverty and increasing health inequalities. Accordingly, there is a pressing need to invest in CVD prevention as a major part of socio-economic development as the burden of non-communicable disease (NCD) will continue to rise in LMICs, disproportionally affecting the poor. The poor have the worst outcomes from NCDs, including CVD, largely because of their inability to access or afford preventative services and ongoing treatments. This calls for a more integrated approach for the detection, prevention and management of CVD in LMICs. In 2005 global health funding per death for HIV/AIDS was $1029 compared with $320 for NCDs (WHO 2005a), indicating that there is a widespread apathy with major health development funds, placing less emphasis in tackling NCDs in LMICs compared to other diseases. Thus, concerted global, regional and local partnerships are pivotal to address this silent epidemic. The United Nations General Assembly convened a high-level meeting on NCDs in New York in September 2011 to take action against this global epidemic. As a result the World Health Organization (WHO) was tasked with delivering a compelling agenda, now enshrined in the *WHO Global Action Plan for the Prevention and Control of NCDs* covering the period 2013–2020. Therefore national governments, policy-makers and international development partners have a key role in ensuring that CVD prevention and control becomes a major part of the health care development agenda.

CVD creates an enormous impact on socio-economic development due to societal and global determinants (Strong et al. 2005; WHO 2005a; Suhrcke et al. 2006) as many of those in the high-risk group are at the peak of their productive and economic activity (Nugent 2008; Alwan and MacLean 2009; Alwan et al. 2010). These determinants include rapid globalisation, unplanned urbanisation, global trade and agricultural policies amongst other things, which ultimately influence an individual's or a society's ability to make healthy choices contributing to its negative impact on social and economic growth in LMICs (Lloyd-Williams et al. 2008). The economic impact in regard to loss of productive years of life and the need to divert scarce resources to tertiary care is substantial. CVD has a multifactorial aetiology with a number of potentially modifiable risk factors. Much of the population attributable risk of CVD is accountable on the basis of nine modifiable traditional risk factors, including smoking, history of hypertension or diabetes, obesity, unhealthy diet, lack of physical activity, excessive alcohol consumption, raised blood lipids and psychosocial factors (Gersh et al. 2010). Eight of these risk factors (excessive alcohol use, tobacco use, high blood pressure, high body mass index (BMI), high cholesterol, high blood glucose, dietary choices and physical inactivity) account for 61% of CVD deaths globally. About 84% of the total global burden of disease they cause occurs in LMICs, with studies showing that alleviating exposure to these eight risk factors would improve global life expectancy by almost five years (WHO 2005b, 2009). Thus further elucidation of the role of these risk factors is important for developing clear and effective strategies for improving global health.

Epidemiological transition

The increasing burden of CVD in LMICs can be largely explained by the epidemiologic transition theory which provided a useful evolutionary framework for understanding changes in disease patterns as a result of demographic factors (ageing and population growth) as well as socio-economic and behavioural changes such as the spread of Western diets and an increase in sedentary lifestyle (Omran 1971; Cappuccio 2004). This highlights that health risk factors are in transition, with an improvement in traditional risks which causes infectious diseases (possibly as a result of improvements in medical care and public health interventions such as vaccinations and the provision of clean water and sanitation targeted to reduce the incidence of infectious diseases). On the other hand factors like urbanisation, globalisation, westernisation and industrialisation result in the emergence of modern risks due to lifestyle changes (e.g. physical inactivity, obesity, other diet-related factors and smoking and alcohol-related risks) that are strong behavioural risk factors and increase the incidence and burden of CVDs in LMICs. The success in the fight against infectious diseases also results in a reduction of infant mortality rates and an increase in life expectancy, resulting in an ageing of the population, but changes in patterns of physical activity and food, alcohol and tobacco consumption predispose this ageing population to the risk of developing CVD. Prolonged survival allows for longer exposure to CVD risk factors and this inevitably results in larger total numbers of CVD cases (Danaei . 2011a, 2011b; Finucane et al. 2011). As a result, many LMICs are faced with a growing added burden from the modern risks factors which increase the incidence of CVD and other chronic NCDs whilst simultaneously dealing with the traditional risks of communicable diseases (known as 'double burden of disease'). Often there is no public health infrastructure or budget to address both communicable and NCDs such as CVD. Currently, these risk factors and measures to deal with the CVD and other chronic diseases epidemic are greatly influenced by political, social, behavioural, environmental and economic determinants, stressing the need for an effective, consolidative multi-sectoral response to deal with the CVD epidemic and help promote socio-economic development in LMICs (WHO 2008).

How to prevent CVD in LMICs?

In most LMICs, awareness of CVD is low, due to technical, human, lack of infrastructure and financial resource constraints which are major impediments to the implementation of cost-effective CVD prevention and control programmes. The rates of detection and treatment of CVD and risk factors reported in many LMICs are critically low, and many people with these diseases have no access to appropriate health care. Lack of information and public awareness means late presentation of most NCD patients in LMICs, making treatment much more expensive. However, prevention and management of CVD risk have been shown to be cost-effective and affordable even in LMICs and should be the main intervention that should be adopted to address this pending epidemic. There is a need to determine disease burden and create awareness in communities on the dangers of CVD which will shift the conventional mode of addressing CVD from tertiary care to primary care and the community with emphasis on risk reduction. This will generate evidence and best practices for cost-effective and long-term community-based strategies for prevention and control of CVD risk factors, creating an effective treatment, lower costs of care and a reduction in the burden of CVD (WHO 2007). Thus intervention at the primary health care level for its prevention and management is a necessity for effective CVD control programmes in these settings at a national level (Reddy 2004). A number of key things must be addressed for an effective implementation of CVD control programmes, including the lack of research capacity, the poor infrastructure of the health care systems, the lack of research work focusing on CVD in these settings that would provide the evidence needed by health care decision-making policy-makers in LMICs to produce highly focused, quality assessed and policy-relevant summaries of research evidence in the field of CVD prevention, management and control. On the same note, government leaders are often slow or even reluctant to acknowledge the need for allocating adequate funding, without jeopardising current and future funding of the prevention and control of communicable diseases, to facilitate local evidence geared towards prevention and management of CVD at the population level. A strategic approach wherein effective primary intervention measures are developed, social, economic and environmental conditions and risk factors are addressed, best practices from other settings in the design of CVD prevention and control strategies are consulted by health policy-makers and evidence-based approaches for interventions for vulnerable groups and populations are adopted, would facilitate the achievement of a structured, integrated programme in CVD prevention (Institute of Medicine (US) Committee on Preventing the Global Epidemic of Cardiovascular Disease: Meeting the Challenges in Developing Countries 2010).

The importance of population-based approach through community-based interventions

As the burden of CVD in LMICs is projected to increase, it is essential to identify and evaluate current effective strategies implemented in CVD prevention and control programmes being adopted in LMICs as it might provide tools for new concerted prevention programmes in these settings. In this issue of the journal, van de Vijver et al. evaluated the effectiveness of community-based interventions for CVD prevention programmes in LMICs to assess their effectiveness of a population-based approach to CVD prevention. A review of the literature was carried out for community-based studies carried out in line with the American Heart Association Framework for public health practice for CVD prevention that were conducted between 1979 and 2008, and published between 1993 and 2011. A total of 26 population-based and high-risk population interventions studies were included (urban or mixed urban and rural setting), that compared intervention groups with non-intervention control groups, before and after the intervention on a number of behavioural outcomes (including tobacco and alcohol use, dietary habits, level of physical activity and salt intake), physical measurements (i.e. waist circumference, weight, systolic and/or diastolic blood pressure, hypertension and BMI), other biomarkers of risk (glucose and HbA1c levels) and the level of awareness, treatment and control of hypertension and diabetes. The outcome of each study was rated in terms of cost-effectiveness, feasibility and training on CVD prevention if this information was available. The aim of the study was to determine which community-based interventions were effective in reducing cardiovascular risk in LMICs at national and regional level. Health promotion using the media and health education as a platform at the national and regional level was mainly used in the population intervention studies, with the end goal of raising knowledge, awareness and healthy behaviour changes at different levels such as diet, exercise, smoking and alcohol use. On the other hand the high-risk population approach focused more on the education of patients, training of health care providers and the implementation of treatment guidelines. Five of these population-based interventions focused on modifying a specific CVD risk factor like salt reduction, healthier diets and exercising. In general, some studies showed a significant reduction of cardiovascular risk ranging from behavioural changes to outcomes like blood pressure, glucose levels or weight and an improved management of risk factors like increased control of hypertension or adherence to medication.

Important insights emerged from the present study. There are promising results from health education and health promotion through media; other means of communication, training of health care providers and the implementation of treatment guidelines, where feasible, are effective; follow-up and adherence are often barriers to an effective delivery of preventive strategies and may vary by age and gender; and several examples around the world confirm the feasibility of these approaches in LMICs. The various constraints that limit the implementation of effective CVD prevention and control measures and the lack of political backing and effective health policies are to be thoroughly addressed. The many challenges that LMICs face in implementing effective prevention and management programmes of CVD are not insurmountable, in preventing the epidemic from reaching its full potential with several affordable, adaptable and feasible multi-disciplinary interventions for prevention being available for adoption in these settings. Major efforts must be made by key stakeholders to direct scarce resources to interventions that are cost-effective, culturally appropriate and sustainable. Accordingly these challenges could be addressed through comprehensive and sustainable approaches, incorporating health education awareness programmes through the media at the population level and implementing preventive measures with health care and treatment with a focus on diet and salt given the fact that they are largely associated with lifestyle factors, training health care staff and implementing treatment guidelines aimed to reduce the prevalence, enable early detection and provide appropriate care and treatment form key elements in successful programmes as shown by the conclusions of this review (van de Vijver et al. 2013). This is in agreement with other studies in the literature.

What to prioritise?

The most cost-effective interventions are tobacco control and salt reduction, and low-cost generic drugs for people at high risk of developing CVD, requiring community involvement for promoting access to services (Asaria et al. 2007). These interventions, if incorporated into population-based interventions, would avert 13.8 million deaths over 10 years in 23 LMICs (Asaria et al. 2007) and promote adherence to prevention protocols. Introducing treatment guidelines that are applicable to an LMIC setting and providing training for health care providers are also an important element in the fight against CVD. Accordingly, it is important to encourage and support active research in LMICs to produce data available to health policy-makers that would justify and increase the financial investments in CVD and possibly the re-evaluation of current health policies in place in LMICs or the development of new effective ones. Reducing salt intake at the population level, including reduction of salt levels in processed foods and food additives, and sustained public education to encourage change in food choices, is an easy way to implement, cost-effective method for preventing, managing and controlling CVD (Gomez and Cappuccio 2005; Cappuccio et al. 2006), making it a financially favourable intervention in LMICs. High salt intake has been shown to cause high blood pressure and to contribute to the incidence of strokes and other cardiovascular events (Strazzullo et al. 2009; Aburto et al. 2013), and a moderate reduction in population salt intake is estimated to lead to a 23% reduction in stroke rates (Cappuccio et al. 2011). It is an easily modifiable environmental factor and it is possible by nutritional education to reduce population blood pressure. This method is particularly effective in reducing the blood pressure of people of African descent as dietary salt is commonly added to the food during cooking or at table (Cappuccio et al. 2006).

These approaches, in turn, need to be underpinned by well-functioning health systems that are able to concurrently address both communicable and NCD. The health care infrastructure in these settings ought to be addressed and strengthened with the necessary political and community support to bring out the required health system reform, with effective monitoring and evaluation, and surveillance systems in place. It is quite evident in the literature that there is a gap in CVD research in LMICs compared to high-income countries (Ebrahim et al. 2013). The fragile research capacity, inadequate financial investment, the language barriers and the exclusion of journals edited in LMICs from a number of online resources are both a consequence and a contributory factor to the widening gap between the health of high-income countries and LMICs, and indicate the need for research capacity building in all areas of NCD policy, advocacy, legislation and strategy (Mendis et al. 2003). Likewise local government and international health partnerships should build commitment, broaden awareness across governments and communities and address constraints faced by the health system. The quote below by the director for the surveillance of NCDs at the WHO forcefully summarises the critical issues related to CVD in LMICs.

> The challenge of the cardiovascular disease epidemic is not whether it will occur at all in the developing countries but whether we respond in time to telescope the transition and avoid the huge burden in young and middle age adults. The question is not whether we can afford to invest in cardiovascular disease prevention in the developing countries, but whether we can afford not to. (Ruth Bonita)

CVD prevention in LMICs is necessary, feasible and affordable. Clearly, the time has now come for action and implementation.

Acknowledgements

The studies on which this article is based have been funded throughout the years by the British Heart Foundation, The Wellcome Trust (060415/Z/00/Z, 069500/Z/02/Z and 072666/Z/03/Z), the EC Research Directorate FP5 (QLK1-CT-2000-00100) and FP7 (HEALTH-F4-2007-201550) and the WHO and the Bupa Foundation (MR-12-002). The publication does not necessarily represent the decisions or the stated policy of WHO, and the designations employed and the presentation of material do not imply the expression of any opinion on the part of WHO.

Haja R. Wurie and Francesco P. Cappuccio

WHO Collaborating Centre for Nutrition, Division of Mental Health & Wellbeing, Warwick Medical School, University of Warwick, Coventry, UK

References

Aburto N. J., A. Ziolkovska, L. Hooper, P. Elliott, F. P. Cappuccio, and J. J. Meerpohl. 2013. "Effect of Lower Sodium Intake on Health Outcomes: Systematic Review and Meta-Analysis." *British Medical Journal.*

Alwan, A., and D. R. MacLean. 2009. "A Review of Non-communicable Disease in Low- and Middle-income Countries." *International Health* 1 (1): 3–9. doi:10.1016/j.inhe.2009.02.003.

Alwan, A., D. R. MacLean, L. M. Riley, E. T. d'Espaignet, C. D. Mathers, G. A. Stevens, and D. Bettcher. 2010. "Monitoring and Surveillance of Chronic Non-communicable Diseases: Progress and Capacity in High-Burden Countries." *Lancet* 376 (9755): 1861–1868. doi:10.1016/S0140-6736(10)61853-3.

Asaria, P., D. Chisholm, C. Mathers, M. Ezzati, and R. Beaglehole. 2007. "Chronic Disease Prevention: Health Effects and Financial Costs of Strategies to Reduce Salt Intake and Control Tobacco Use." *Lancet* 370 (9604): 2044–2053. doi:10.1016/S0140-6736(07)61698-5.

Cappuccio, F. P. 2004. "Commentary: Epidemiological Transition, Migration, and Cardiovascular Disease." *International Journal of Epidemiology* 33 (2): 387–388. doi:10.1093/ije/dyh091.

Cappuccio, F. P., S. Capewell, P. Lincoln, and K. McPherson. 2011. "Policy Options to Reduce Population Salt Intake." *British Medical Journal* 343: 402–405. http://dx.doi.org/10.1136bmj.d4995.

Cappuccio, F. P., S. M. Kerry, F. B. Micah, J. Plange-Rhule, and J. B. Eastwood. 2006. "A Community Programme to Reduce Salt Intake and Blood Pressure in Ghana." *BMC Public Health* 6 (1): 13. doi:10.1186/1471-2458-6-13.

Danaei, G., M. M. Finucane, J. K. Lin, G. M. Singh, C. J. Paciorek, M. J. Cowan, F. Farzadfar, et al. 2011a. "National, Regional, and Global Trends in Systolic Blood Pressure Since 1980: Systematic Analysis of Health Examination Surveys And Epidemiological Studies With 786 Country-Years and 5.4 Million Participants." *Lancet* 377 (9765): 568–577. doi:10.1016/S0140-6736(10)62036-3.

Danaei, G., M. M. Finucane, Y. Lu, G. M. Singh, M. J. Cowan, C. J. Paciorek, J. K. Lin, et al. 2011b. "National, Regional, and Global Trends in Fasting Plasma Glucose and Diabetes Prevalence since 1980: Systematic Analysis of Health Examination Surveys and Epidemiological Studies with 370 Country-Years and 2.7 Million Participants." *Lancet* 378 (9785): 31–40. doi:10.1016/S0140-6736(11)60679-X.

Ebrahim, S., N. Pearce, L. Smeeth, J. P. Casas, S. Jaffar, and P. Piot. 2013. "Tackling Non-Communicable Diseases in Low- and Middle-Income countries: Is the Evidence from High-Income Countries All We Need? *PLoS Medicine* 10 (1): 1001377. doi:10.1371/journal.pmed.1001377.

Finucane, M. M., G. A. Stevens, M. J. Cowan, G. Danaei, J. K. Lin, C. J. Paciorek, G. M. Singh, et al. 2011. "National, Regional, and Global Trends in Body-Mass Index Since 1980: Systematic Analysis of Health Examination Surveys and Epidemiological Studies with 960 Country-Years and 9.1 Million Participants." *Lancet* 377 (9765): 557–567. doi:10.1016/S0140-6736(10)62037-5.

Gersh, B. J., K. Sliwa, B. M. Mayosi, and S. Yusuf. 2010. "Novel Therapeutic Concepts: The Epidemic of Cardiovascular Disease in the Developing World: Global Implications." *European Heart Journal* 31 (6): 642–648. doi:10.1093/eurheartj/ehq030.

Gomez, G. B., and F. P. Cappuccio. 2005. "Dietary Salt and Disease Prevention: A Global Perspective." *Current Medicinal Chemistry – Immunology, Endocrine & Metabolic Agents* 5: 13–20. www.ingentaconnect.com/content/ben/cmciema/2005/00000005/00000001/art00003.

Institute of Medicine (US). Committee on Preventing the Global Epidemic of Cardiovascular Disease: Meeting the Challenges in Developing Countries. 2010. *Promoting Cardiovascular Health in the Developing World: A Critical Challenge to Achieve Global Health*. Edited by Fuster, V., and B. B. Kelly. Washington, DC: National Academies Press.

Lloyd-Williams, F., M. O'Flaherty, M. Mwatsama, C. Birt, R. Ireland, and S. Capewell. 2008. "Estimating the Cardiovascular Mortality Burden Attributable to the European Common Agricultural Policy on Dietary Saturated Fats." *Bulletin of the World Health Organization* 86 (7): 535–541. http://www.who.int/bulletin/volumes/86/7/08-053728.pdf.

Mendis, S., D. Yach, R. Bengoa, D. Narvaez, and X. Zhang. 2003. "Research Gap in Cardiovascular Disease in Developing Countries." *Lancet* 361 (9376): 2246–2247. doi:10.1016/S0140-6736(03)13753-1.

Nugent, R. 2008. "Chronic Diseases in Developing Countries: Health and Economic Burdens." *Annals of the New York Academy of Sciences* 1136 (1): 70–79. doi:10.1196/annals.1425.027.

Omran, A. R. 1971. "The Epidemiologic Transition. A Theory of the Epidemiology of Population Change." *The Milbank Memorial Fund Quarterly* 49 (4): 509–538. doi:10.2307/3349375.

Reddy, K. S. 2004. "Cardiovascular Disease in Non-Western Countries." *New England Journal of Medicine* 350 (24): 2438–2440. www.nejm.org/doi/full/10.1056/NEJMp048024.

Strazzullo, P., L. D'Elia, N.-B. Kandala, and F. P. Cappuccio. 2009. "Salt Intake, Stroke and Cardiovascular Disease: A Meta-Analysis of Prospective Studies." *British Medical Journal* 339: b4567. doi:10.1136/bmj.b4567.

Strong, K., C. Mathers, S. Leeder, and R. Beaglehole. 2005. "Preventing Chronic Diseases: How Many Lives Can We Save? *Lancet* 366 (9496): 1578–1582. doi:10.1016/S0140-6736(05)67341-2.

Suhrcke, M., M. McKee, D. Stuckler, R. Sauto Arce, S. Tsolova, and J. Mortensen. 2006. "The Contribution of Health to the Economy in the European Union." *Public Health* 120 (11): 994–1001. doi:10.1016/j.puhe.2006.08.011.

van de Vijver, S., S. Oti, J. Addo, A. de Graft-Aikins, and C. Agyemang. 2013. "Review of Community-Based Interventions for Prevention of Cardiovascular Diseases in Low- and Middle-income Countries." *Ethnicity & Health*. doi:10.1080/13557858.2012.754409

WHO. 2005a. *Preventing Chronic Diseases: A Vital Investment*. Geneva: The World Health Organization.

WHO. 2005b. *The Role of CVD Risk Factors (WHO Global InfoBase Team). The SuRF Report 2. Surveillance of Chronic Disease Risk Factors: Country-Level Data and Comparable Estimates.* Geneva: World Health Organization.

WHO. 2007. *Prevention of Cardiovascular Disease: Guidelines for Assessment and Management of Total Cardiovascular Risk*. Geneva: World Health Organization.

WHO. 2008. *Commission on Social Determinants of Health. Closing the Gap in a Generation: Health Equity through Action on the Social Determinants of Health.* Geneva: World Health Organization.

WHO. 2009. *Global Health Risks: Mortality and Burden of Disease Attributable to Selected Major Risks.* Geneva: World Health Organization.

WHO. 2011. *Global Status Report on Noncommunicable Diseases 2010*. Geneva: World Health Organization.

Ethnicity and cardiovascular health research: pushing the boundaries by including comparison populations in the countries of origin

Charles Agyemang[a], Ama de-Graft Aikins[b] and Raj Bhopal[c]

[a]Department of Public Health, Academic Medical Centre, University of Amsterdam, Amsterdam, The Netherlands; [b]Regional Institute for Population Studies, University of Ghana, Legon, Ghana; [c]Edinburgh Ethnicity and Health Research Group, Public Health Sciences Section, Centre for Population Health Sciences, University of Edinburgh, Edinburgh, UK

Chronic diseases such as cardiovascular diseases (CVD) are major health problems in most ethnic minority and migrant populations living in high income countries. By the same token, CVD is a looming threat that is creating a double burden in most of the countries where these populations originate from. The causes of the rising burden are unclear, but they are likely to be multifaceted. Traditionally, ethnicity and health research have mostly concentrated on comparing the health of ethnic minority groups with the majority populations of the countries in which they live. This is an important area of research which illuminates ethnic inequalities in health. However, a few studies on international comparisons show that a lot can be learned from comparing similar ethnic groups living in different industrialised countries. Equally, comparing ethnic minority and migrant populations to similar populations in their countries of origin will generate new knowledge about factors that predispose them to poor health outcomes. Thus, to make progress in the field of ethnicity and health research, we need a new conceptual framework that simultaneously studies migrant/ethnic groups in the country of settlement, in similar countries of settlement, and in the countries of ancestral origin. Such studies need to go beyond the commonest design of cross-sectional studies to include more cohort studies, interventions and linkage studies. This article discusses (1) the burden of CVD in ethnic minority and migrant populations; (2) approaches to understanding predisposing factors; and (3) application of the results to give insight into the potential threats that their countries of origin are likely to face.

A note on terminology relating to ethnicity

There is no consensus on appropriate terms for the scientific study of health by ethnicity. By ethnicity we mean the group a person belongs to as a result of a mix of cultural factors including language, diet, religion and ancestry. We have also followed principles in the glossary by Bhopal (2004). For example, in Europe the term ethnic minority group usually refers to minority populations of non-European origin. We use it this way here. There is no universally accepted definition of migrant. The term migrant is usually used to refer to persons and family members, moving to another country or region to better their material or social conditions and to improve the prospects for themselves or their family (IOM, *Glossary on migration*, 2004). For this article, we use the terms 'migrants' to refer to the individuals born in low-and middle-income countries (LMIC) but residing in the high income countries of Europe and North America. The term 'local born' is used to refer to residents born in the migrants' host country.

Introduction

Increasing globalisation and technology have made the modern world more interconnected and interdependent. The effects of these shared connections and dependencies have included increasing international migration (Gushulak 2010). Consequently, ethnic minority and migrant populations form significant and rising proportions of the industrialised nations' populations. Changing populations pose important challenges for epidemiology, public health and clinical care.

One of the most important health problems affecting ethnic minority and migrant populations in industrialised countries today is cardiovascular diseases (CVD) (Bos *et al.* 2005, Gill *et al.* 2007, Wild *et al.* 2007, Agyemang *et al.* 2009a). CVD and risk factors are also a looming threat in most low- and middle-income countries (LMIC; Abegunde *et al.* 2007, Mensah 2008) where most minority populations in Europe originate from. The causes of the increasing burden of CVD in ethnic minority groups as well as in LMIC are complex (Godfrey and Julien 2005, de-Graft Aikins *et al.* 2010). The increasing burden of CVD in LMIC is mainly driven by globalisation, economic development, urbanisation and the increasing adoption of the lifestyles associated with such changes (Godfrey and Julien 2005). These changes in lifestyles include reduced physical activity, tobacco use and adoption of diets with a high proportion of saturated fat and sugars. Although the burden of CVD in LMIC is apparent, the institutional response to prevention and control is limited. Many decades of neglect of non-communicable diseases (NCD) in LMIC have created a situation whereby many LMIC still lack data and policy on CVD (WHO 2011). Where there are policies, they are often non-functional because of the general lack of political will and the widespread apathy by the major health development funds and bilateral aid programmes in tackling CVD in LMIC (Nugent and Feigl 2010). National capacity for CVD prevention and control is weak and the institutional response to capacity building has not kept pace with the epidemiological transition (Beaglehole and Yach 2003). Very little (i.e., <3%) of the global development assistance for health, goes to prevention and control of chronic non-communicable diseases in LMIC (Nugent and Feigl 2010). The need to address the NCD burden in LMIC is gaining credence. This was aptly highlighted in the 2011 meeting of the general assembly of the United Nations addressing NCD as an important epidemic of our times (http://www.un.org/en/ga/president/65/issues/ncdiseases.shtml).

Given the general lack of information particularly on the local determinants of CVD in many LMIC (Fuster and Kelly 2010), data on ethnic minority groups and migrant populations originating from LMIC but living in high income countries of Europe and North America may provide useful insights into both the potential future CVD threat to these countries and increasing understanding of factors that predispose these populations to the high risk of CVD.

This article discusses (1) the burden of CVD in ethnic minority and migrant populations; (2) approaches to understanding of predisposing factors; and (3) application of the results to give insight into the potential threats that their countries of origin are likely to face. Examples will be drawn from the recent international comparative studies including the European Commission (EC) funded projects on CVD and risk factors among ethnic minority and migrant populations.

The burden of CVD in ethnic minority and migrant populations

Ethnic minority and migrant populations in Europe have different CVD health outcomes than the local born populations (Bos *et al.* 2005, Gill *et al.* 2007, Wild *et al.* 2007, Agyemang *et al.* 2009a). In many cases they have worse outcomes, although in some instances their outcomes are better. The relative differences in CVD rates between the locally born and the migrant population are largely dependent on ethnic background, type of CVD and risk factor, country of residence and the length of stay in the host country. South-Asian born (i.e., India, Pakistani, Bangladeshi and Sri Lanka) people who migrated to England and Wales, for example, have higher mortality from both stroke and ischemic heart diseases (IHD) than the England and Wales national average (Gill *et al.* 2007, Wild *et al.* 2007). People born in the West Indies/Caribbean or West Africa but residing in England and Wales have lower mortality from IHD, but higher mortality from stroke than the England and Wales national average (Gill *et al.* 2007, Wild *et al.* 2007). Similar consistent findings have also been reported among South Asian and African populations living in other European countries (Bos *et al.* 2004, Regidor *et al.* 2008, 2009). In addition, Turkish-born and Polish-born populations also have a higher risk of death from circulatory diseases than the locally born European populations (Bhopal *et al.* 2011). By contrast, low CVD mortality rates have been reported in some migrant populations in a few studies (Bos *et al.* 2004, Gray *et al.* 2007, Regidor *et al.* 2008, 2009).

The prevalence of CVD risk factors also differ among ethnic groups. Essential hypertension, a major risk factor for stroke, is highly prevalent among West African descent populations living in Europe and North America (Agyemang and Bhopal 2002, 2003, Hajjar and Kotchen 2003, Agyemang *et al.* 2006) and appears to be a major contributor to the elevated stroke risk observed among West African diaspora populations. The prevalence of hypertension in West African descent populations is 2–4 times higher than in White people (Agyemang and Bhopal 2003, Hajjar and Kotchen 2003, Agyemang *et al.* 2006). For example, in the SUNSET study, the African-Surinamese men and women living in the Netherlands were twice and almost four times, respectively, more likely than their locally born White-Dutch counterparts to have hypertension (Agyemang *et al.* 2005, 2006). The little available evidence seems to suggest that West Africans who have migrated directly from West Africa might even be at higher risk of hypertension than other African origin populations. In our recent pilot study among recent Ghanaian migrants in Amsterdam, the Netherlands, the prevalence of hypertension was 54% in men and 56% in women (Agyemang *et al.* 2012); far above the prevalence rates reported among African-Surinamese in the Netherlands (Agyemang *et al.* 2005, 2006) and African-Americans in the USA (Hajjar and Kotchen 2003). High blood pressure levels also appears to be common in South Asian populations living in the Netherlands as compared to the European-Dutch people, but the levels were mostly lower in South Asian populations particularly in the Bangladeshi population in the UK compared to the UK generational population (Agyemang and Bhopal 2002, Agyemang *et al.* 2005). The prevalence of hypertension was shown to be lower among Turkish and Moroccan ethnic groups than in European-Dutch people living in the Netherlands (Agyemang *et al.* 2006).

Generally, data on type II diabetes among ethnic minority and migrant populations are still limited (Oldroyd *et al.* 2005). However, the limited data suggest that most ethnic minority and migrant populations are disproportionately affected by diabetes compared with the host populations. The prevalence of type II diabetes, for example, is about three to five times greater in some groups compared with the host European populations (Oldroyd *et al.* 2005, Ujcic-Voortman *et al.* 2009). They also develop diabetes at a younger age; and they have higher morbidity and mortality from diabetes and related complications such as CVD than European host populations (Uitewaal *et al.* 2004, Oldroyd *et al.* 2005, Ujcic-Voortman *et al.* 2009). A recent report by Ujcic-Voortman *et al.* (2009) shows that the typical age of onset of type II diabetes in Turkish and Moroccan ethnic groups were one and two decades younger than in European-Dutch populations, respectively (Ujcic-Voortman *et al.* 2009). These differences corroborate with the higher type II diabetes mortality among ethnic minority groups relative to the European locally born populations (Mather *et al.* 1998, Vandenheede *et al.* 2012). Adiposity, a major risk factor for diabetes and other CVD risk factors, is also a major problem in ethnic minority groups particularly in women compared to the European host populations (Misra and Ganda 2007, Agyemang *et al.* 2009b, Fernandez *et al.* 2011, Ujcic-Voortman *et al.* 2012).

The burden of CVD in migrants' countries of origin

Whilst CVD is a major health burden in most ethnic minority groups living in high income countries of Europe and North America; it is also increasingly becoming a looming threat that is creating a double burden in LMIC where many of these populations originate (Unwin *et al.* 2001, Abegunde *et al.* 2007, Gaziano 2007, Mensah 2008, WHO 2011). In 2005, about 80% of all CVD deaths occurred in LMIC (Mathers and Loncar 2006). In addition, the global burden of disease projection suggests that the burden of CVD will continue to rise. It has been estimated that almost 23.6 million people will die annually from CVD by 2030, with approximately 85% happening in LMIC (Mathers and Loncar 2006). CVD affect people from all walks of life including urban and rural populations, rich and poor, old and young. Even in sub-Saharan Africa where infectious diseases are still the overall leading cause of death, CVD is the second leading killer overall and the leading cause of death among adults aged 30 years and older, who are in their most productive years of life (Gaziano 2005, 2007). Over the next few years the sub-Saharan Africa is projected to experience one of the largest increases in death rates from non-communicable chronic diseases (Gaziano 2007). CVDs are, therefore, no longer syndromes of wealthy societies; they are becoming just as dominant in LMIC.

The main drivers of the rising CVD in LMIC are the increasing prevalence of major risk factors such as hypertension, diabetes, obesity and smoking. The prevalence rates of diabetes and hypertension in many LMIC countries far exceed those reported in high-income countries (Kearney *et al.* 2005, Shaw *et al.* 2010). The global estimates also indicate that the increases in the prevalence of hypertension and diabetes will be higher in LMIC than in high-income countries (Kearney *et al.* 2005, Shaw *et al.* 2010). For instance, Shaw *et al.* (2010) estimates indicate that for LMIC, adult diabetes numbers are likely to increase by 69% from 2010 to 2030, compared to 20% for high-income countries. Kearney *et al.* (2005) estimates also show that the number of people with hypertension in LMIC will increase by 80% in 2025, compared with 24% in high income countries. Similarly, LMIC are projected to have a much larger proportional increase in the number of overweight and obese individuals than high income countries between 2005 and 2030 (Kelly *et al.* 2008). Time trend analyses, for example, show that the prevalence of obesity in urban West Africa has more than doubled over the last 15 years (Abubakari *et al.* 2008).

The rising levels of CVD in LMIC clearly reflects the changing lifestyle such as consumption of energy-dense foods and refined sugars complemented by less energy-demanding jobs particularly in the urban centres, which are linked to structural factors such as urbanisation and increasing globalisation of the food market (WHO/ FAO 2003, WHO 2005, Prentice 2006).

The burden is further compounded by weak health systems that are unable to cope with the double burden of CVD and infectious diseases (Beaglehole *et al.* 2007).

Explanations for the ethnic differences in CVD

The reasons for the high risk of CVD and prevalence of risk factors as well as its complications in ethnic groups and migrant populations are difficult to explain. Several factors have been proposed including low socio-economic position (SEP), unhealthy behaviour following migration (for example, physical inactivity, regular smoking and poor eating habits), and genetic factors (Rotimi and Cooper 1995, McKeigue 1997, Nazroo 1998, Misra and Ganda 2007, Agyemang *et al.* 2009c, Palmer *et al.* 2011). Low SEP has been one of the most widely discussed factors for the ethnic inequalities in health (Nazroo 1998, Stronks and Kunst 2009). This is probably due to the fact that many ethnic minority groups are often socio-economically disadvantaged relative to the majority populations; and low SEP may also influence migration related lifestyle changes such as dietary and sedentary behaviours. Poor SEP, for example, may limit ethnic minority groups' ability to afford healthy foods and to engage in leisure time physical activity. Genetic factors have also been well discussed as potential factors in explaining ethnic differences in health (McKeigue 1997). However, the contribution of genetic factors to the ethnic differences in health is often very small and the results are often difficult to replicate (Cooper and Zhu 2001, Cruickshank *et al.* 2001, Cooper 2003, Li *et al.* 2006). For example, sequence variations in the human α_2 adrenergic receptor genes (ADRA2A and ADRA2C) were implicated as a cause of hypertension in African-American subjects (Lockette *et al.* 1995, Neumeister *et al.* 2005). From a stratified random population sample of 1767 subjects, however, Li *et al.* (2006) found no association of either variant with hypertension in African-Americans.

Favourable health outcomes in some ethnic minority and migrant populations relative to the host populations observed in some European and North American countries, especially in all-cause mortality and cancers (Wanner *et al.* 1997, Razum *et al.* 1998, Singh and Hiatt 2006) are often interpreted as the 'healthy migrant effect'. The 'healthy migrant effect' theory proposes that the better health outcome of migrant populations is due to the fact that the healthiest people in the country of origin migrate. Poor health is commonly attributed to factors such as low SEP or genetics, and better health is attributed to 'healthy migrant effect'. These two explanations may be applied in the same ethnic group within a country, and often times in the same study. For example, in one Canadian study (Sheth *et al.* 1999), the low cancer mortality in South Asian descent population relative to the European Canadian was interpreted as a possible 'healthy migrant effect'. By contrast, the higher rates of death from IHD and diabetes within the same South-Asian group was suggested to be related to factors such as dietary factors, exposure to environmental smoke from tobacco and increased genetic susceptibility. The commonality of cancer and CVD risk factors, however, undermines the usefulness of such general explanations.

Such general explanations may have slowed down progress in understanding ethnic difference in health. This is because such explanations may dissuade researchers from looking for explanations. Undoubtedly factors such as low SEP may have a profound effect on adverse CVD outcomes among ethnic minority groups; however, it does not entirely explain ethnic differences in health (Bindraban *et al.* 2008, Bos *et al.* 2005). This may partly due to the fact that the assessment of SEP across ethnic minority and migrant populations is complex, which makes it difficult to correctly estimate the extent to which SEP contributes to ethnic differences in health due to residual confounding (Kaufman *et al.* 1997). The SEP also seems to act differently across different ethnic groups in relation to health outcome (Bhopal *et al.* 2002, Nierkens *et al.* 2006, Agyemang *et al.* 2010a). Besides, not all ethnic minority groups are economically disadvantaged; the Indian people in the UK today are not socio-economically disadvantaged yet they have worse CVD outcomes than the general population in the UK. In addition, it is not only healthy people who migrate, but people also migrate for several reasons including political instability, economic, family unification, famine and for reasons of poor health. Consequently, the need to move beyond these dominating explanatory models is increasingly being recognised (Nazroo 2003, Sniderman *et al.* 2007, Agyemang *et al.* 2010b, Spallek *et al.* 2011). In the last few years, several explanatory factors have been proposed for explaining ethnic inequalities in health including psychosocial factors such as discrimination (Nazroo 2003), adipose tissue overflow hypothesis for increased metabolic disorders in South Asian descent populations (Sniderman *et al.* 2007), and the role of national context on CVD (Agyemang *et al.* 2010b). Discrimination, for example, has been suggested to be a focal element of larger societal disparities which generates ethnic inequalities in health (Karlsen and Nazroo 2002). Socio-political structures and conditions that create ethnic harmony or ethnic disharmony may differ between countries and subsequently affect ethnic minority and migrant populations' CVD health outcomes in different ways. It has been emphasised that the challenge to political culture by migration not only lies in the cultural difference that ethnic minority groups bring into the political community, but also for a large part in the willingness and ability of a society's majority population to tolerate or reconcile such difference with the principles of liberal democracy (Duyvené de Wit and Koopmans 2005).

Approaches for studying ethnic inequalities in health

One of the most important decisions in assessing the health status of ethnic minority and migrant populations is the population against which the ethnic minority and migrant populations are being compared. Most of the current research on ethnicity and health is confined (both conceptually and empirically) to the countries in which these populations live. Although country-specific studies are crucial in assessing ethnic inequalities in health, extending ethnicity and health research across national borders will further enrich our understanding of ethnic inequalities in health. A few studies have shown the power of this (Marmot *et al.* 1975, Bhatnagar *et al.* 1995, Nazroo *et al.* 2007, Agyemang *et al.* 2010b, Bhopal *et al.* 2011), and we need to do more to advance on these types of studies.

There are two other important approaches in which the health status of ethnic minority and migrant populations can be assessed across national boundaries: (1) comparison of a similar ethnic or migrant population living in different locations (Nazroo *et al.* 2007, Agyemang *et al.* 2010b, Bhopal *et al.* 2011); and (2) comparison of an ethnic group or migrant population with similar populations in the country of origin who did not migrate (Marmot *et al.* 1975, Bhatnagar *et al.* 1995, Agyemang *et al.* 2009b). The comparison of the similar ethnic minority groups across different industrialised countries is more recent development than the comparison with country of origin populations. Each of these approaches can reveal important aspects of how the migratory process and its consequences affect and influence the health of ethnic minority and migrant populations. Knowledge on health outcomes that are directly linked to the migration process will allow for the most effective and appropriate use of interventions, efforts and investment to improve and promote the health of these populations (Gushulak 2010). Comparison between ethnic minority and migrant population with the same population in the country of origin will also reveal the future CVD threats in the country of origin as many of these countries continue to westernise.

Comparison of similar ethnic minority or migrant populations living in different countries

Comparing similar ethnic minority or migrant groups living in different industrialised countries offers an important alternative approach in assessing ethnic inequalities in health (Nazroo *et al.* 2007, Agyemang *et al.* 2010b, Bhopal *et al.* 2011). This is particularly relevant because the industrialised countries themselves differ. Even among rich nations in Europe and North America there are clear differences in CVD health outcomes (Wolf-Maier *et al.* 2004, Cooper *et al.* 2005). The potential causes of the health inequalities between industrialised countries have been well debated. The effect of relative deprivation, for example, is thought to be a potential underlying factor between differences in health across countries (Wilkinson 1996, Wilkinson and Pickett 2007, Marmot *et al.* 2012). Evidence seems to suggest that mortality tends to be lower in countries where income differences are smaller than countries where income differences are larger, even after average incomes, absolute poverty, and a number of other socio-economic factors have been adjusted for (Wilkinson 1996). Besides, the local situation of ethnic minority and migrant populations such as socio-economic development of the groups, race relations and access to health care and preventive services may vary greatly among countries (Fernandes and Miguel 2009, Agyemang *et al.* 2010b). These differential contexts can influence health behaviour, psychosocial stress and health care use among ethnic minority and migrant groups, and subsequently lead to differences in CVD health outcomes between similar populations living in different countries. Whilst several factors for example, the local circumstances, genetic predispositions and early life circumstances may influence the health of the ethnic minority and migrant groups, the health status of the local reference population will ultimately determine the relative health standing of the ethnic minority and migrant groups within the country in which they live. For example, health status of ethnic minority and migrant groups may seem better than the local reference population, not because they are healthy, but because the reference local population is particularly unhealthy, and vice versa. We refer to this as a 'migrant pond effect' or 'migrant context effect'. This 'migrant pond effect' is to some extent similar to the 'frog-pond effect' theory in educational research (Alicke *et al.* 2010). This 'frog-pond effect' theory suggests that for the same frog, the effect of being in a pond filled with big frogs is different than being in a pond filled with small frogs. Thus, for the same ethnic minority or migrant group, the interpretation of their health status will depend on the relative health standing of the local reference population.

An example of studies comparing similar ethnic minority or migrant populations living in different countries is demonstrated in a recent comparative analysis of CVD risk factors between English and Dutch ethnic groups by Agyemang *et al.* (2010b, 2011a, 2011b). The authors used similar surveys from the UK (the Health Survey for England and the Newcastle Heart Project) and the Netherlands (the SUNSET study) to explore the role of national context on CVD risk factors among South Asian and African Caribbean populations living in these two countries. They found, for example, that the prevalence of smoking was higher in Dutch South Asian and African-Caribbean populations than in their English South Asian and African-Caribbean counterparts in England (Agyemang *et al.* 2011a; Figure 1).

The prevalence of smoking initiation was also higher and smoking cessation was lower in the Dutch South Asian and African-Caribbean populations than in their English equivalent counterparts. These differences reflected a similar pattern of differences between the White-Dutch and White-English people. These results suggest that the particular circumstances in the host country, such as the ways in which anti-smoking policies have been implemented, may strongly modify CVD risks of ethnic minority and migrant groups living in these countries.

Another example is the study of Bhopal *et al.* (2011) where they compared circulatory disease mortality in the same country of birth group across European countries. They found substantial between-country differences. In general, the lowest mortality rates occurred in France although people born outside France had high rates of circulatory diseases compared with those who were born in France. Despite these inequalities within France, ethnic minority groups born outside France but living in France also enjoy relatively low rates of circulatory diseases compared to those in the same country of birth groups residing in other countries. For example, Poland born men had a total circulatory mortality rate of 630/100,000 in Denmark and 499/100,000 in England/Wales compared to 154/100,000 in France. A similarly varied pattern was observed in women for example, Poland born had a rate of 265/100,000 in Denmark, 126/100,000 in England and 54/100,000 in France. These

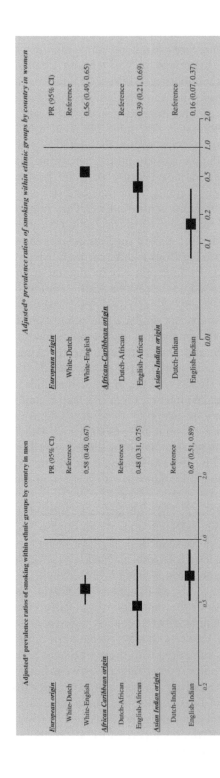

Figure 1. Prevalence ratios of smoking between Dutch and English ethnic groups (Adapted from Agyemang *et al.* 2011a). *Adjusted for age, survey year, SES and length of stay.

findings suggest that disease outcomes may be influenced by the local context, including health care, diagnostic methods and coding, social and economic standing, stress, lifestyle, migration history, social circumstances and health prior to migration or other environmental factors (Bhopal *et al.* 2011).

These kinds of studies can generate relevant information to develop healthcare and public health interventions, and also generate hypotheses into the causes, consequences and control of CVD among ethnic minority and migrant populations (Bhopal 2009). These data are, however, limited and mainly based on cross-sectional studies, which have numerous methodological limitations. Hence more studies including cohort and longitudinal studies are needed in this area of research.

Comparison between migrant populations with populations in country of origin

Many LMIC are experiencing rapid changes in lifestyle associated with rapid urbanisation. The rapid rises of CVD in migration populations' living in high income countries gives indications of how the burden will unfold if immediate and appropriate actions are not taken. Given the rising prevalence of CVD in migrant populations as well as in their countries' of origin, research approaches that can simultaneously give insight into the high risk of CVD in migrant populations and the populations in their countries of origin might be a useful and cost effective way of addressing the problem. Such studies also provide opportunities to assess the health impact of different selection of migrants to different countries. A limited number of studies have compared CVD and its risk factors of migrant populations to populations of their countries of origin although the main interests were on the migrant populations rather than the populations in the countries of origin. One well-known example was the study on men of Japanese ancestry aged 45–69 living in Japan, Hawaii and California (Marmot *et al.* 1975). The age-adjusted prevalence rate for definite coronary heart disease (CHD) was lower in Japanese men living in Japan (5.3/1000) than those living in California (10.8/1000). For definite plus possible CHD the rates were lower in Japanese men living in Japan (25.4/1000) than Japanese men living Hawaii (34.7/1000) and California (44.6/1000). The rate of angina pectoris and pain of possible myocardial infarction, determined by questionnaire, showed a similar gradient. In another study, migrants from the Indian subcontinent of Punjabi origin living in West London, the UK were compared with their siblings living in the Punjab in India (Bhatnager *et al.* 1995). The authors found that Punjabi people living in West London had a greater body mass index, systolic blood pressure, serum cholesterol, apolipoprotein B, lower high-density lipoprotein cholesterol and higher fasting blood glucose than their siblings in the Punjab. Another example of studies comparing migrant populations with their country of origin is demonstrated by the recent comparative analysis of overweight and obesity among Ghanaian migrants living in Amsterdam, the Netherlands, with compatriots living in urban and rural Ghana. The authors found a marked increasing gradient in the prevalence of overweight and obesity from rural Ghana to Amsterdam (Figure 2). In a logistic regression analysis adjusting for age and education, Ghanaian migrants living in Amsterdam were 10 times more likely than Ghanaians living rural Ghana to be overweight and obese (Agyemang *et al.* 2009b).

These kinds of comparative studies have a huge potential not only for ethnic minority and migrant populations, but also for the country from which they have

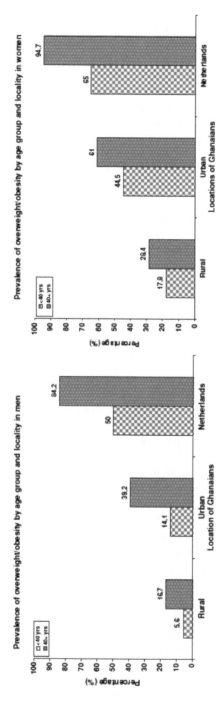

Figure 2. Prevalence of overweight/obesity among Ghanaian migrants and their compatriots in their rural and urban Ghana (reproduced from Agyemang et al. (2009b) with permission from Cambridge University Press.

migrated from. For ethnic minority and migrant populations, it gives indications of how exposure to different environmental circumstances might influence health outcomes. For the country of origin, the rapid increase of CVD following migration to industrialised countries gives a clear indication of the vulnerability of the population left behind. The influence of internal migration has been illustrated in studies that have shown poorer CVD health outcomes in urban communities than in their rural peers in LMIC (Agyemang *et al.* 2006, Addo *et al.* 2007, Gupta and Misra 2007). The continuing trend of urbanisation, as is expected in LMIC is likely to lead to a situation where the NCD risk in populations living in their country of origin would ultimately resemble that of their compatriots living abroad. Comparisons between the migrants and non-migrants in the countries of origin also provide an opportunity to identify specific lifestyle changes following migration that might predispose migrant populations to a high risk of diseases. Such information is critically important for public health and policy response to addressing the CVD burden in ethnic minority and migrant groups as well as in their countries' of origin (Fernandes and Miguel 2009). Studies on lifestyle changes following migration are, however, limited. Given the potential benefits of such information both to migrating populations as well as their countries of origins, such studies are a priority. Careful standardisation of the study protocols including appropriate comparable populations in the country of origin is key to success of this approach. The importance of such studies is highlighted by the recent EC initiative on gene–environmental interactions on obesity and diabetes among migrant populations in the EU (2012). Below we describe briefly one of the EC funded projects (i.e., RODAM) to demonstrate how such studies can be carried out.

RODAM study

RODAM (an acronym for Research on Obesity and Diabetes among African Migrants) is a multi-centre project (www.ro-dam.eu). The main aim of the RODAM project is to understand the reasons for the high prevalence of type II diabetes and obesity in African migrants by studying the complex interplay between social circumstances, lifestyle, biochemistry and (epi)genetics and their relative contributions to the high risk of type II diabetes and obesity; and to identify specific risk factors within these broad categories to guide intervention programmes and provide a basis for improving diagnosis and treatment. A conceptual model for the RODAM project is presented in Figure 3.

The conceptual model shows that following migration, migrants may be exposed to varied national contexts such as different opportunities for socio-economic development, availability of food, health systems and policies and cultural traditions; and these differences may influence their health behaviour, physical and psychosocial stress and subsequently lead to differences in obesity and type II diabetes risks. In particular, the influence of migration on the relative role of identified risk factors for obesity and diabetes will be estimated. In addition, epigenetic programming may contribute to the increased susceptibility of migrants towards obesity and diabetes. Therefore, changes in the epigenetic pattern (DNA methylation and expression) upon migration will be examined, and investigated with respect to a differential importance of risk alleles between African migrants in Europe and their counterparts in Africa.

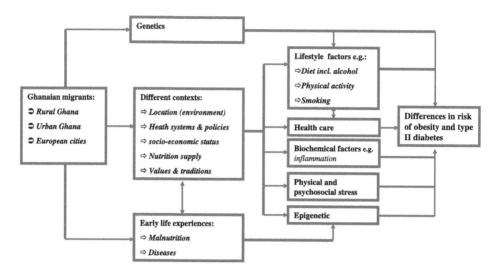

Adapted from Agyemang C et al. 2011. *Epidemiology*, 22 (4), 563-7.

Figure 3. A conceptual model for the RODAM project (Adapted from Agyemang *et al.* 2011b).

Assessing social circumstances, lifestyle and genetic influence on health among ethnic minority and migrant populations requires a homogenous migrant population and a well standardised approach. Therefore, we focus on one relatively homogenous African group (i.e., Ghanaians) living in three European countries (Germany, the Netherlands and UK) and rural and Urban Ghana. In a multi-centre study, 6250 Ghanaians (1250 per site) aged $\geq$ 25 years will be recruited in rural and urban Ghana, Germany, the Netherlands and UK. Data collection will be identical at all sites following standard operating procedures and applying standardised tools. Strictly standardised methods will ensure the comparability of data/samples obtained at the various recruitment sites. The set of the study also provides important opportunity to follow up the study participants over time in various recruitment sites.

Results from studies such as RODAM will be highly relevant for both migrants as well as their compatriots in the country of origin. This will allow us to draw conclusions on the magnitude of the problem and deduce the attributable risk of migration from rural to urban as well as migration to Europe. The findings on the influence of migration (from Africa to Europe) will help health care providers and health policy stakeholders to better understand and predict comparable developments in other African populations and in other parts. The impact of such studies is also likely to be greater than studies based on individual countries.

Conclusion

In conclusion, comparative studies on similar ethnic minority and migrant populations living in different industrialised countries as well as in their countries' of origin, provide promising avenues in advancing our understanding of the underlying disease processes in both migrant populations and the populations in their countries of origin. Such studies may also provide important opportunities to move ethnic and health research forward into uncharted territories such as the contribution of epigenetics to the increased susceptibility of migrant population towards CVD. Undoubtedly, such studies will require more resources and careful standardisation of the study methods than studying ethnic or migrant populations within a country; and partnerships between LMIC and industrialised nations in order to obtain comparable data. Nevertheless, with the recent rising burden of CVD in LMIC where many migrant populations originate from, research that can simultaneously provide relevant information for the migrating populations as well as non-migrating populations might be a cost effective way of gaining insights into the problem. For ethnic minority and migrant populations, such information might give insights into how exposure to different environmental circumstances might influence health outcomes. For their compatriots in LMIC, the rapid increase of CVD following migration to industrialised countries gives a clear indication of the potential future CVD threat as these countries continue to westernise, and suggests the need for strengthening research capacity in these countries.

Key messages

(1) To make progress in ethnicity and health research we need a new conceptual framework that simultaneously study migrant/ethnic groups in the country of settlement, in similar countries of settlement and in the countries of ancestral origin.
(2) Such studies need to go beyond the commonest design of cross-sectional studies, to include more cohort studies, interventions and linkage studies.
(3) Such studies should include more detailed information so that we can move towards potential explanations beyond description.

Acknowledgements

We thank Dr Ank de Jonge, Dr Anton Kunst, Dr Mary Nicolaou and Dr Erik Beune for their useful suggestions. We are also very grateful to the four anonymous reviewers who provided excellent comments, which helped to further improve our article.

References

Abegunde, D.O., *et al.*, 2007. The burden and costs of chronic diseases in low-income and middle-income countries. *Lancet*, 370 (9603), 1929–1938.

Abubakari, A.R., *et al.*, 2008. Prevalence and time trends in obesity among adult West African populations: a meta-analysis. *Obesity Reviews*, 9 (4), 297–311.

Addo, J., *et al.*, 2007. Hypertension in sub-Saharan Africa: a systematic review. *Hypertension*, 50, 1012–1018.

Agyemang, C. and Bhopal, R.S., 2002. Is the blood pressure of South Asian adults in the UK higher or lower than that in European white adults? A review of cross-sectional data. *Journal of Human Hypertension*, 16 (11), 739–751.

Agyemang, C. and Bhopal, R., 2003. Is the blood pressure of people from African origin adults in the UK higher or lower than that in European origin white people? A review of cross-sectional data. *Journal of Human Hypertension*, 17, 523–534.

Agyemang, C., *et al.*, 2005. Prevalence, awareness, treatment, and control of hypertension among Black Surinamese, South Asian Surinamese and White Dutch in Amsterdam, The Netherlands: the SUNSET study. *Journal of Hypertension*, 23, 1971–1977.

Agyemang, C., *et al.*, 2006. Prevalence and management of hypertension among Turkish, Moroccan and native Dutch ethnic groups in Amsterdam, the Netherlands: The Amsterdam Health Monitor Survey. *Journal of Hypertension*, 24 (11), 2169–2176.

Agyemang, C., *et al.*, 2009a. Risk of death after first admission for cardiovascular diseases by country of birth in the Netherlands – a nationwide record linked retrospective cohort study. *Heart*, 95, 747–753.

Agyemang, C., *et al.*, 2009b. Overweight and obesity among Ghanaian residents in The Netherlands: how do they weigh against their urban and rural counterparts in Ghana? *Public Health Nutrition*, 12 (7), 909–916.

Agyemang, C., *et al.*, 2009c. Cardiovascular disease, diabetes and established risk factors among populations of sub-Saharan African descent in Europe: a literature review. *Globalization and Health*, 5, 7.

Agyemang, C., *et al.*, 2010a. Educational inequalities in metabolic syndrome vary by ethnic group: evidence from the SUNSET study. *International Journal of Cardiology*, 141 (3), 266–274.

Agyemang, C., *et al.*, 2010b. Ethnic inequalities in health: does it matter where you have migrated to? *Ethnicity and Health*, 15 (3), 216–218.

Agyemang, C., *et al.*, 2011a. A cross-national comparative study of smoking prevalence and cessation between English and Dutch South Asian and African origin populations: the role of national context. *Nicotine and Tobacco Research*, 12 (6), 557–566.

Agyemang, C., *et al.*, 2011b. Diabetes prevalence in populations of South Asian Indian and African origins: a comparison of England and the Netherlands. *Epidemiology*, 22 (4), 563–567.

Agyemang, C., *et al.*, 2012. Prevalence, awareness, treatment, and control of hypertension among Ghanaian population in Amsterdam, the Netherlands: the GHAIA study. *European Journal of Preventive Cardiology*. doi:10.1177/2047487312451540

Alicke, M.D., Zell, E., and Bloom, D.L., 2010. Mere categorization and the frog-pond effect. *Psychological Science*, 21 (2), 174–177.

Beaglehole, R. and Yach, D., 2003. Globalisation and the prevention and control of non-communicable disease: the neglected chronic diseases of adults. *Lancet*, 362 (9387), 903–908.

Beaglehole, R., *et al.*, 2007. On behalf of the Chronic Disease Action Group. Prevention of chronic disease: a call to action. *Lancet*, 370, 2152–2157.

Bhatnagar, D., *et al.*, 1995. Coronary risk factors in people from the Indian subcontinent living in west London and their siblings in India. *Lancet*, 345 (8947), 405–409.

Bhopal, R., 2004. Glossary of terms relating to ethnicity and race: for reflection and debate. *Journal of Epidemiology and Community Health*, 58, 441–445.

Bhopal, R., 2009. Chronic diseases in Europe's migrant and ethnic minorities: challenges, solutions and a vision. *European Journal of Public Health*, 19, 140–143.

Bhopal, R., *et al.*, 2002. Ethnic and socio-economic inequalities in coronary heart disease, diabetes and risk factors in Europeans and South Asians. *Journal of Public Health Medicine*, 24, 95–105.

Bhopal, R.S., *et al.*, 2011. Mortality from circulatory diseases by specific country of birth across six European countries: test of concept. *European Journal of Public Health*. [Epub ahead of print]

Bindraban, N.R., *et al.*, 2008. Prevalence of diabetes mellitus and the performance of a risk score among Hindustani Surinamese, African Surinamese and ethnic Dutch: a cross-sectional population-based study. *BMC Public Health*, 8, 271.

Bos, V., *et al.*, 2004. Ethnic inequalities in age- and cause-specific mortality in The Netherlands. *International Journal of Epidemiology*, 33 (5), 1112–1119.

Bos, V., *et al.*, 2005. Socioeconomic inequalities in mortality within ethnic groups in the Netherlands, 1995–2000. *Journal of Epidemiology and Community Health*, 59 (4), 329–335.

Cooper, R.S., 2003. Race, genes, and health – new wine in old bottles? *International Journal of Epidemiology*, 32 (1), 23–25.

Cooper, R.S., *et al.*, 2005. An international comparative study of blood pressure in populations of European vs. African descent. *BMC Medicine*, 3, 2.

Cooper, R.S. and Zhu, X., 2001. Racial differences and the genetics of hypertension. *Current Hypertension Reports*, 3, 19–24.

Cruickshank, J.K., *et al.*, 2001. Sick genes, sick individuals or sick populations with chronic disease? The emergence of diabetes and high blood pressure in African-origin populations. *International Journal of Epidemiology*, 30, 111–117.

de-Graft Aikins, A., *et al.*, 2010. Tackling Africa's chronic disease burden: from the local to the global. *Globalization and Health*, 6, 5.

Duyvené de Wit, T. and Koopmans, R., 2005. The integration of ethnic minorities into political culture: The Netherlands, Germany and Great Britain compared. *Acta Politica*, 40, 50–73.

European Commission, 2012. DIABESITY – A World-Wide Challenge. Towards a global initiative on gene-environment interactions in diabetes/obesity in specific populations. Available from: http://ec.europa.eu/research/health/events-12_en.html [Accessed January 2012].

Fernandes, A. and Miguel, J.P., eds., 2009. *Health and migration in the European Union: better health for all in an inclusive society.* Lisbon: Instituto Nacional de Saude Doutor Ricardo Jorge.

Fernandez, R., Miranda, C., and Everett, B., 2011. Prevalence of obesity among migrant Asian Indians: a systematic review and meta-analysis. *International Journal of Evidence-Based Healthcare*, 9 (4), 420–428.

Fuster, V. and Kelly, B.B., 2010. *Promoting cardiovascular health in the developing world.* Washington, DC: National Academies Press.

Gaziano, T.A., 2005. Cardiovascular disease in the developing world and its cost-effective management. *Circulation*, 112, 3547–3553.

Gaziano, T.A., 2007. Reducing the growing burden of cardiovascular disease in the developing world. *Health Affairs (Millwood)*, 26 (1), 13–24.

Gill, P.S., *et al.*, 2007. Black and minority ethnic groups. *In*: A. Stevens, J. Raftery, and J. Mant, eds. *Health care needs assessment: the epidemiologically based needs assessment reviews.* Abingdon, UK: Radcliffe Medical Press, 227–239.

Godfrey, R. and Julien, M., 2005. Urbanisation and health. *Clinical Medicine*, 5 (2), 137–141.

Gray, L., Harding, S., and Reid, A., 2007. Evidence of divergence with duration of residence in circulatory disease mortality in migrants to Australia. *European Journal of Public Health*, 17 (6), 550–554.

Gupta, R. and Misra, A., 2007. Type 2 diabetes in India: regional disparities. *British Journal of Diabetes and Vascular Disease*, 7, 12–16.

Gushulak, B., 2010. Monitoring migrants' health. *In*: Report of a global consultation, Madrid, Spain 3–5 March 2010. *Health of migrants – The way forward.* Geneva: World Health Organization, 28–42.

Hajjar, I. and Kotchen, T.A., 2003. Trends in prevalence, awareness, treatment, and control of hypertension in the United States, 1988–2000. *JAMA*, 290, 199–206.

Karlsen, S. and Nazroo, J.Y., 2002. Relation between racial discrimination, social class, and health among ethnic minority groups. *American Journal of Public Health*, 92, 624–631.

Kaufman, J.S., Cooper, R.S., and McGee, D.L., 1997. Socioeconomic status and health in blacks and whites: the problem of residual confounding and the resiliency of race. *Epidemiology*, 8, 621–628.

Kearney, P.M., *et al.*, 2005. Global burden of hypertension: analysis of worldwide data. *Lancet*, 365 (9455), 217–223.

Kelly, T., *et al.*, 2008. Global burden of obesity in 2005 and projections to 2030. *International Journal of Obesity (London)*, 32 (9), 1431–1437.

Li, J.L., *et al.*, 2006. Do allelic variants in alpha2A and alpha2C adrenergic receptors predispose to hypertension in blacks? *Hypertension*, 47, 1140–1146.

Lockette, W., *et al.*, 1995. Alpha 2-adrenergic receptor gene polymorphism and hypertension in blacks. *American Journal of Hypertension*, 8 (4 Pt 1), 390–394.

Marmot, M.G., *et al.*, 1975. Epidemiologic studies of coronary heart disease and stroke in Japanese men living in Japan, Hawaii and California: prevalence of coronary and hypertensive heart disease and associated risk factors. *American Journal of Epidemiology*, 102, 514–525.

Marmot, M., *et al.*, 2012. Building of the global movement for health equity: from Santiago to Rio and beyond. *Lancet*, 379 (9811), 181–188.

Mather, H.M., Chaturvedi, N., and Fuller, J.H., 1998. Mortality and morbidity from diabetes in South Asians and Europeans: 11-year follow-up of the Southall Diabetes Survey, London, UK. *Diabetic Medicine*, 15 (1), 53–59.

Mathers, C.D. and Loncar, D., 2006. Projections of global mortality and burden of disease from 2002 to 2030. *PLoS Medicine*, 3, 2011–2030.

McKeigue, P.M., 1997. Mapping genes underlying ethnic differences in disease risk by linkage disequilibrium in recently admixed populations. *American Journal of Human Genetics*, 60, 188–196.

Mensah, G.A., 2008. Ischaemic heart disease in Africa. *Heart*, 94, 836–843.

Misra, A. and Ganda, O.P., 2007. Migration and its impact on adiposity and type 2 diabetes. *Nutrition*, 23 (9), 696–708.

Nazroo, J., 1998. Genetic, cultural or socio-economic vulnerability? Explaining ethnic inequalities in health. *Sociology of Health and Illness*, 20, 710–730.

Nazroo, J., 2003. The structuring of ethnic inequalities in health: economic position, racial discrimination and racism. *American Journal of Public Health*, 93, 277–284.

Nazroo, J., *et al.*, 2007. The Black diaspora and health inequalities in the US and England: does where you go and how you get there make a difference? *Sociology of Health and Illness*, 29 (6), 811–830.

Neumeister, A., *et al.*, 2005. Sympathoneural and adrenomedullary functional effects of alpha2C-adrenoreceptor gene polymorphism in healthy humans. *Pharmacogenetics and Genomics*, 15, 143–149.

Nierkens, V., *et al.*, 2006. Smoking in immigrants: do socioeconomic gradients follow the pattern expected from the tobacco epidemic? *Tobacco Control*, 15, 385–391.

Nugent, R. and Feigl, A., 2010. *Where have all the donors gone? Scarce donor funding for non-communicable diseases. Center for Global Development*. Working Paper 228. November, Washington.

Oldroyd, J., *et al.*, 2005. Diabetes and ethnic minorities. *Postgraduate Medical Journal*, 81, 486–490.

Palmer, N.D., *et al.*, 2011. Resequencing and analysis of variation in the TCF7L2 gene in African Americans suggests that SNP rs7903146 is the causal diabetes susceptibility variant. *Diabetes*, 60, 662–668.

Prentice, A.M., 2006. The emerging epidemic of obesity in developing countries. *International Journal of Epidemiology*, 35, 93–99.

Razum, O., *et al.*, 1998. Low overall mortality of Turkish residents in Germany persists and extends into second generation: merely a healthy migrant effect? *Tropical Medicine and International Health*, 3, 297–303.

Regidor, E., *et al.*, 2008. Heterogeneity in cause-specific mortality according to birthplace in immigrant men residing in Madrid, Spain. *Annals of Epidemiology*, 8 (8), 605–613.

Regidor, E., *et al.*, 2009. Mortality from cardiovascular diseases in immigrants residing in Madrid. *Medicina Clínica (Barc)*, 132 (16), 621–624.

Rotimi, C. and Cooper, R., 1995. Familial resemblance for anthropometric measurements and relative fat distribution among African Americans. *International Journal of Obesity and Related Metabolic Disorders*, 19, 875–880.

Shaw, J.E., Sicree, R.A., and Zimmet, P.Z., 2010. Global estimates of the prevalence of diabetes for 2010 and 2030. *Diabetes Research and Clinical Practice*, 87, 4–14.

Sheth, T., *et al.*, 1999. Cardiovascular and cancer mortality among Canadians of European, south Asian and Chinese origin from 1979 to 1993: an analysis of 1.2 million deaths. *CMAJ*, 161 (2), 132–138.

Singh, G.K. and Hiatt, R.A., 2006. Trends and disparities in socioeconomic and behavioural characteristics, life expectancy, and cause-specific mortality of native-born and foreign-born populations in the United States, 1979–2003. *International Journal of Epidemiology*, 35, 903–919.

Sniderman, A.D., *et al.*, 2007. Why might South Asians be so susceptible to central obesity and its atherogenic consequences? The adipose tissue overflow hypothesis. *International Journal of Epidemiology*, 36 (1), 220–225.

Spallek, J., Zeeb, H., and Razum, O., 2011. What do we have to know from migrants' past exposures to understand their health status? A life course approach. *Emerging Themes in Epidemiology*, 8 (1), 6.

Stronks, K. and Kunst, A.E., 2009. The complex interrelationship between ethnic and socio-economic inequalities in health. *Journal of Public Health (Oxford)*, 31 (3), 324–325.

Uitewaal, P.J., *et al.*, 2004. Prevalence of type 2 diabetes mellitus, other cardiovascular risk factors, and cardiovascular disease in Turkish and Moroccan immigrants in North West Europe: a systematic review. *Preventive Medicine*, 39 (6), 1068–1076.

Ujcic-Voortman, J.K., *et al.*, 2009. Diabetes prevalence and risk factors among ethnic minorities. *European Journal of Public Health*, 19 (5), 511–515.

Ujcic-Voortman, J.K., *et al.*, 2012. Obesity and cardiovascular disease risk among Turkish and Moroccan migrant groups in Europe: a systematic review. *Obesity Reviews*, 13 (1), 2–16.

Unwin, N., *et al.*, 2001. Noncommunicable diseases in sub-Saharan Africa: where do they feature in the health research agenda? *Bulletin of the World Health Organisation*, 79 (10), 947–953.

Vandenheede, H., *et al.*, 2012. Migrant mortality from diabetes mellitus across Europe: the importance of socio-economic change. *European Journal of Epidemiology*, 27 (2), 109–117.

Wanner, P., Bouchardy, C., and Khlat, M., 1997. Causes de deècés des immigrés en France 1979–1985. *Migrations Santé*, 91, 9–38.

WHO, 2005. *Preventing chronic disease. A vital investment*. Geneva: WHO.

WHO, 2011. Cardiovascular diseases. Fact sheet number 317. Available from: http://www.who.int/mediacentre/factsheets/fs317/en/index.html [Accessed December 2011].

WHO/FAO, 2003. *Diet, nutrition and the prevention of chronic diseases: report of a joint WHO/FAO expert Consultation*. Geneva: WHO.

Wild, S.H., *et al.*, 2007. Mortality from all causes and circulatory disease by country of birth in England and Wales 2001–2003. *Journal of Public Health (Oxford)*, 29, 191–198.

Wilkinson, R.G., 1996. *Unhealthy societies: the afflictions of inequality*. London: Routledge.

Wilkinson, R.G. and Pickett, K.E., 2007. The problems of relative deprivation: why some societies do better than others. *Social Science and Medicine*, 65 (9), 1965–1978.

Wolf-Maier, K., *et al.*, 2004. Hypertension treatment and control in five European countries, Canada, and the United States. *Hypertension*, 43, 10–17.

'A chronic disease is a disease which keeps coming back ... it is like the flu': chronic disease risk perception and explanatory models among French- and Swahili-speaking African migrants

Maxwell Cooper[a], Seeromanie Harding[b], Kenneth Mullen[c] and Catherine O'Donnell[a]

[a]General Practice and Primary Care, Institute of Health & Wellbeing, College of Medical, Veterinary and Life Sciences, University of Glasgow, Glasgow, UK; [b]Social and Public Health Sciences Unit, Medical Research Council, University of Glasgow, Glasgow, UK; [c]School of Medicine, College of Medical, Veterinary and Life Sciences, University of Glasgow, Glasgow, UK

Background. African migrants to the West are at increased risk of hypertensive related diseases and certain cancers compared with other ethnic groups. Little is known about their awareness of this risk or knowledge of associated risk factors.
Objectives. To explore African migrants' perceptions of chronic disease risk, risk factors and underlying explanatory models.
Design. In-depth interviews with 19 Africans from French- or Swahili-speaking countries living in Glasgow were conducted. Interviews were transcribed and 10 translated (3 Swahili and 7 French). Analysis was informed by a grounded theory approach.
Results. Narratives suggested low awareness of chronic disease risk among participants. Africans reported a positive outlook on life that discouraged thought about future sickness. Infectious diseases were considered the dominant health threat for African migrants, mainly HIV but also TB and 'flu'. Chronic diseases were sometimes described as contagious. Explanatory models of chronic disease included bodily/dietary imbalance, stress/exertion, heredity/predisposition and food contamination. Cancer was feared but not considered a major threat. Cancer was considered more common in Europe than Africa and attributed to chemical contamination from fertilisers, food preservatives and industrial pollution. Evidence cited for these chemicals was rapid livestock/vegetable production, large size of livestock (e.g., fish), softness of meat and flavourless food. Chemicals were reported to circulate silently inside the body and cancer to form in the part where they deposit, sometimes years later. Cardiovascular diseases were described in terms of acute symptoms that required short-term medication. Confidentiality concerns were reported to prevent discussion of chronic disease between Africans.
Conclusion. This study suggests a need to improve chronic disease health literacy among African migrants to promote engagement with preventive behaviours. This should build on not only participants' existing knowledge of disease causation and risk factors but also their self-reliance in the pursuit of a healthy lifestyle and desire to retain cultural knowledge and practice.

Background

Non-communicable chronic diseases are now the greatest cause of death in the world (Yach *et al.* 2004). This global epidemiological transition has been linked with adoption of less healthy diets, physical inactivity, tobacco use, urbanisation, increased life expectancy and poverty (World Health Organisation 2005). This epidemic has particular relevance to Africa and to African migrants because over the next decade the continent is expected to face the greatest rise in mortality from these conditions (Graft Aikins *et al.* 2010). Already in Africa there is an increasing incidence of cancer (Parkin *et al.* 2008), ischaemic heart disease (Mensah 2008), diabetes (Levitt 2008) and obesity (Dalal *et al.* 2011) and the lifetime risk of dying from cancer amongst women is almost double that of developed countries (Parkin *et al.* 2008).

Africans are a significant migrant group to the UK. Between 2002 and 2009 the Black African population of England and Wales grew 6.2% per year with significant migration from the African Commonwealth countries, as well as Somalia, Eritrea and the Democratic Republic of Congo (Office for National Statistics 2011). In 2009, 47,405 Africans and their dependents entered the UK, of whom 30,945 came as students and 16,460 on work visas (Home Office 2010). In addition, there is a substantial African asylum seeker and refugee population in the UK: in 2008 there were 7585 asylum applications from Zimbabwe, Eritrea, Somalia and Nigeria (Information Centre about Asylum and Refugees 2009). Over the past 10 years many asylum seekers have been moved from the South East of England to other UK cities (including Glasgow) as part of the UK Borders Agency dispersal programme. These changing patterns of migration mean that many British clinicians will be asked to provide care for African migrants.

African migrants to Europe are known to experience increased mortality and morbidity from major chronic diseases such as circulatory diseases, including stroke and diabetes (Harding *et al.* 2008, Vandenheede *et al.* 2012). Major cancers such as breast, colon and prostate cancers are also leading causes of cancer deaths (Harding *et al.* 2009). Higher rates of hypertension have also been reported in people of African descent in the UK (Agyemang and Bhopal 2003) and there is evidence that Africans who migrate have higher blood pressure and greater cardiovascular risk than their counterparts who do not (Dominguez *et al.* 2009).

There is a large body of evidence for the social patterning of ethnic differences in chronic disease mortality and morbidity in the UK (Davey-Smith *et al.* 2000), in Europe (Harding *et al.* 2008, Vandenheede *et al.* 2012) and the USA (Krieger 2000). Such differences may be attributed to a range of factors, including the structural conditions under which migrants live as well as aspects of individual behaviour and agency (Factor *et al.* 2011). Observed increased risk of and mortality in people of African descent, for example from prostatic cancer, may, therefore, be based on factors such as socio-economic status, diet, and/or differences in disease detection (Kheirandish and Chinegwundoh 2011). Indeed, studies of cancer beliefs amongst migrants to the UK point to the impact of migration on health-related beliefs and behaviours that influence disease risk as people adapt to the new socio-economic and cultural context of their host country (Scanlon *et al.* 2006, Bache *et al.* 2012). Migrant studies thus provide insight into the contextual influences on the retention of and change in beliefs about health and well-being and can inform the development of appropriate interventions.

To counter the chronic disease epidemic an expanded role for primary care services and community based interventions has been advocated in order to address more effectively both prevention and treatment (Allotey *et al.* 2011). Nevertheless, even where health care systems are orientated towards chronic disease management major challenges exist to providing care for migrant groups. First, migrants tend to use health care services for acute problems rather than for prevention (Mullen *et al.* 2007). Second, migrants – including Africans – do not always understand the General Practitioner's (GP) role, may have difficulty adapting to a patient-focused consultation style and report discordant and unmet expectations of GP consultations (O'Donnell *et al.* 2007, 2008). Such divergence may occur around health beliefs, treatment expectations and compliance with medication (Pavlish *et al.* 2010). Central to this are the lay beliefs and explanatory models that underpin the way individuals and groups perceive health and illness.

Lay health beliefs and explanatory models of disease

Lay beliefs are key to understanding different groups' health-seeking behaviour and attitudes towards preventative care. People's beliefs about chronic disease are shaped by its uncertain course, unlimited duration, alternating periods of crisis and remission, and – at times – asymptomatic nature (Scandlyn 2000). One theoretical approach to examining health beliefs is Kleinman's explanatory models of illnesses. This considers the informal notions held by patients, families or practitioners to account for the nature, cause, reason and treatment for an illness (Kleinman 1988, Kleinman and Benson 2006). These models are not necessarily the same as the general beliefs about health held by a given society and individuals may provide different explanations depending on whom they are speaking to (Helman 2007). Indeed, clinicians are often unaware of their patients' explanatory models, especially those with lower educational levels (Helman 1985). Increasing cultural diversity has led to calls to improve the quality of clinical care for minority ethnic groups by promoting the cultural competence of practitioners, in particular communication skills to explore explanatory models and to elicit what is really at stake for patients in the lived experience of their illness (Kleinman and Benson 2006).

Chronic disease management of conditions such as hypertension requires early diagnosis and adherence to lifestyle modifications and/or pharmacological treatments. There is a growing interest, therefore, in how best to promote adherence in the long-term management of chronic conditions in developing nations and in migrants from these countries. This is important amongst Africans because chronicity of disease may not be recognised as a concept by some African societies (Aikins *et al.* 2010). Similarly, African migrants have been found to emphasise symptoms above underlying diagnostic causes for their problems and that symptoms themselves thus come to account for illness (Pavlish *et al.* 2010).

Lay and patient knowledge of major chronic diseases in parts of Africa is considered to be poor and health beliefs are rooted in sociocultural knowledge systems (Aikins *et al.* 2010). Studies in Ghana have examined beliefs about chronic disease causation. Diabetics were found to use a number of explanations for their condition, including: high sugar diets, heredity, physiological imbalance, toxic foods and spiritual disruption (witchcraft and malevolent social actions) (Aikins 2005). Similarly, cardiovascular disease has been attributed by church members in Ghana to a variety of causes, including stress, an unhealthy diet, advanced age and lack of physical activity (Abanilla *et al.* 2011).

Another study compared explanatory models for hypertension among Ghanaians, African-Surinamese and native Dutch hypertensive patients in Amsterdam (Beune *et al.* 2006). Ghanaians and African-Surinamese perceived hypertension as a disease with immediate effects resulting mainly from stress as well as migration-related factors such as adapting to dietary and climate change. Many participants felt a return to their homeland could cure their hypertension and few associated hypertension with obesity, despite many being overweight. It was also noted that some Ghanaians held reservations about sharing their diagnosis with other community members as hypertension was perceived as a sign of domestic problems or an inability to fulfil social obligations.

In the UK, a qualitative study of African and Black Caribbean origin cancer survivors in London suggested a pessimistic view of cancer outcomes and only some knowledge of risk factors, based on diet, alcohol intake, travel history, place of residence and smoking status (Bache *et al.* in press). Cancer was believed to result from complex and diverse factors, again including stress, as well as genetic and divine causes

There is, thus, a need to explore and document chronic disease beliefs and explanatory models, particularly in the context of African migrants. Whilst health beliefs of African-Americans have been studied in depth, little is known about chronic disease risk perception and health beliefs among African migrants in the UK. This paper seeks, therefore, to explore and understand health beliefs in a sample of African migrants living in the West of Scotland.

Method

A qualitative approach was chosen as this is considered particularly suitable for exploring in depth the subtle and sensitive nature of health beliefs. Individual in-depth interviews were conducted with 19 Africans to explore their experience of accessing health care. During the early interviews, Africans were asked which diseases they felt vulnerable to. This led to the emergence of chronic disease risk awareness as an important issue, which was then followed up in greater depth in later interviews. In addition to risk perceptions, later interviews were modified to use Kleinman's theory of explanatory models (Kleinman 1988, Kleinman and Benson 2006) to explore participants' beliefs about the causes, nature and consequences of common chronic diseases and obesity.

Participants

A decision was made to focus on French- and Swahili-speaking African migrants, as these were the languages spoken by the lead researcher (M.C.). Participants were recruited from community organisations, in particular two protestant churches and five African societies based on language or country of origin. A process of onward chain sampling ('snowballing') from initial contacts was employed to facilitate the identification of other, potential respondents (Faugier and Sargeant 1997).

A sampling frame was initially devised to seek maximum diversity in terms of age, gender and religion (i.e., Christian and Muslim traditions) of participants. A target of 24 participants was planned as it was anticipated that data saturation (i.e., when no new themes or issues are raised) would be obtained with such a sample. Initially new participants with similar characteristics were accepted in order to facilitate onward chain sampling. This was also because experience had shown that recruitment might not be straightforward (O'Donnell *et al.* 2007). However, data saturation was reached earlier and, along with a recognition of the length of time required for recruitment, transcription and translation by M.C., the study was curtailed after a total of 19 Africans had been reached. This included a range of participants with the notable exception of Muslim males. Nine primary participants were interviewed and onward 'snowball' recruitment resulted in four chains of one additional participant and one of six additional participants.

Conduct of interviews

An interview schedule was developed based on knowledge of the literature and discussion with medical colleagues and members of African community organisations. Seven interviews were conducted in French, three in Swahili and the rest in English. As many participants were multilingual, interviews often contained words or phrases in the three study languages. Interviews lasted from 34 to 82 minutes (mean = 67 minutes) and were conducted at a time and venue chosen by the participant, including their home, Glasgow University teaching rooms and cafes in the city. Signed consent was obtained prior to interviewing. Africans were given £15 for participating. Ethical approval was granted by the Glasgow University Medical Faculty Ethics Committee.

Translation and data analysis

Interviews were translated by the lead investigator who has experience of conducting qualitative research in French and Swahili in Africa. The accuracy and cultural appropriateness of the translations was assessed by asking native speakers to review randomly selected sections of interview transcriptions. In addition, the translation of quotations selected for this paper were reviewed by and discussed with native African speakers of Swahili and French in order to consider alternative interpretations of the data. Interview transcripts were imported into the NVivo software package to facilitate data coding and analysis. A grounded theory approach was used to inform data analysis, with constant comparison across interviews (Glaser and Strauss 1967) and across key variables such as gender and educational attainment. Following reading and rereading of the transcripts, codes were applied to portions of the text by MC. These were then reviewed and re-ordered into thematic categories. A sample of interviews was also coded by KM and COD. Emerging codes and themes were reviewed in data clinics, where the three coders discussed the identified codes and themes, allowing discrepancies to be reviewed and agreement on coding reached. The final coding framework was then applied to all the interviews. Quotations were selected to illustrate particular points. While seeking to preserve anonymity, quotations include reference to the participant number gender, and age as well as the original language(s) of the quotation used (e.g., 3F 30–39 French).

Results

Nineteen participants were interviewed, of whom nine were women. Apart from three Muslim females all participants were from Christian traditions. Participants were from a broad range of African countries, including both Congo republics, Burundi, Rwanda, Somalia and Kenya. Additional demographic details of the study group are contained in Table 1. Participant health status was not directly sought during recruitment; however, three patients volunteered that they had hypertension (6 and 19), diabetes (6) or asthma (15).

In addition to perceptions of disease risk and beliefs about chronicity and medication adherence, this study identified the following explanatory models: bodily/dietary imbalance, stress/exertion, heredity/predisposition and food contamination with chemicals. These findings – as well participants' beliefs about obesity in the development of chronic disease – are presented below in turn.

Africans' perception of chronic disease risk

Early interviews examined Africans' experiences of consulting doctors in the UK National Health Service. During these, a lack of awareness of chronic disease risk

Table 1. Participant characteristics.

	Age	Religion	Languages (main language of interview given first)	Area of origin	Age of leaving education	Years in UK	Immigration status
1F	25–29	C	Eng/Sw	EA	17	5–10	R
2F	30–39	C	Eng/Sw/OA	EA	17	5–10	MWS
3F	30–39	C	Fr/Eng/OA/OE	Congo	27	5–10	MWS
4F	40–49	C	Fr/Eng/OA	Congo	22	5–10	R
5F	50–59	M	Sw/Eng/OA	EA	21	5–10	R
6F	60–69	C	Fr/OA	Congo	17	5–10	R
7M	20–25	C	Eng/Sw/OA	EA	Still in education	5–10	MWS
8F	30–39	C	Eng/Sw/OA	EA	21	10–15	R
9M	30–39	C	Eng/OA/Sw	EA	24	2–5	MWS
10M	18–24	C	Eng/Fr/Sw	Congo	Still in Education	10–15	R
11F	40–49	M	Swa/Eng	EA	0	5–10	R
12M	30–39	C	Eng/Fr/OA	Francophone West Africa	29	2–5	MWS
13M	30–39	C	Fr/Sw/Eng/OA	Congo	25	5–10	R
14F	30–39	M	Sw/Eng	EA	11	10–15	R
15M	30–39	C	Eng/Fr/Sw//OA	EA	24	10–15	R
16M	40–49	C	Fr/OA/Eng	Congo	25	5–10	R
17M	40–49	C	Fr/Eng/OA	Congo	27	10–15	R
18M	50–59	C	Fr/Eng/OA	Congo	c25	5–10	R
19M	50–59	C	Fr/OE/Eng/OA	Congo	c25	5–10	R

EA = Eastern Africa (Somalia/Tanzania/Uganda/Rwanda/Burundi); Congo = Democratic Republic of the Congo/Republic of Congo, OA = Other African language(s); OE = Other European languages, R = refugee; MWS = Migrant worker/student visa.

became apparent, even among participants with higher levels of education. Many appeared not to be worried about future illness and this was attributed to a focus on symptomatic conditions and a belief in serious disease as a phenomenon that affects other people:

> [Africans are not worried] apart from what they are [already] suffering.... There's nothing people are worried of catching, nobody, I have never heard of anybody thinking about cancer. People think that cancer is maybe somebody else's disease...[laughter]... but not theirs...and you know such things...people are positive. (1 F 25–29 English)

When specifically questioned about major health threats facing African migrants, no participants without an existing chronic disease diagnosis identified cardiac disease, hypertensive disease or diabetes as important threats. Despite most having resided in the UK for 5 years or more, participants tended to talk about infectious and communicable diseases, for example, HIV, tuberculosis, 'flu', sexually transmitted diseases, colds and what was described as 'high fever.' This tendency to consider infectious over non-communicable, chronic disease was underlined by one participant who reported that for lung problems: 'I have always thought of an infection, tuberculosis [rather] than cancer' (17M 40–49 French).

The predominance of the infectious disease model appeared to influence the language participants used to describe chronic conditions. It was notable that some French speaking participants voluntarily described chronic diseases in terms of being 'caught.' This verb was used most commonly for cancer, but also for heart disease, diabetes and hypertension For one participant, transmission was suggested by his attempt to explain diabetes: 'how to prevent diabetes from coming or from penetrating my body? I do not know what it is due to, what transports it, or is it the food, or is it the alcohol?' (16M 40–49 French). For another, it was even reported that Africans might avoid a diabetic 'thinking perhaps it is a contagious disease' (18M 50–59 French).

Amongst healthy participants the only chronic condition that was offered as a threat was cancer. Cancer was frequently recognised as something to be feared and was viewed as incurable. There was also a notion of lack of control over its causation: 'I think everyone is scared of getting cancer – but anyone can' (2F 30–40 English). One participant simplified cancer to internal and external forms: 'there's that cancer disease of the skin and cancer inside the body' (14F 30–39 Swahili). Others, however, recognised that cancer can affect many different parts of, and organs in, the body: 'I know that there are prostate cancers, there are breast cancers, there are stomach cancers, there are cancers in the arms, there are cancers that come in all types' (13M 30–39 French).

When asked, most participants volunteered at least one explanation for cancer, although one struggled to find an explanation:

> like my friend who died of liver cancer he wasn't a heavy drinker, he wasn't someone who drank a lot. You know you are talking about someone who has four or five beers a weekend but he had liver cancer. I really don't understand, it is something up to this day, I don't understand how it happened. (7M 20–25 English)

However, no one suggested that Africans were at any greater risk of developing certain cancers than Europeans. Indeed, a commonly reported observation was that cancer was significantly more common in Europe than Africa: 'in our place [in Africa] there is not a lot of cancer, here there is a lot, but where does that come from, things in the food?' (6F 60–70 French). Indeed, cancer was described as 'a European disease' (17M 40–49 French).

While some participants considered this observation to be correct, a few recognised the issue of under-diagnosis in Africa: 'but now is when I understand that it is only the rich people who could afford to go for scans' (7M 20–25 English). Only once was this perceived difference accounted for in terms of specific risk factors associated with a 'luxurious life': cancer was reported to be more common in Western 'celebrities' due to 'cosmetic products' and 'frequent artificial suntans' (17M 40–49 French).

When confronted with the suggestion that Africans were at increased risk of certain chronic conditions there was widespread surprise: 'I could believe you as a scientist but just looking at [it] like that, I don't think so' (18M 50–59 French). It was reported that the African community was 'not sufficiently informed' about chronic diseases and that Africans only 'learn by going [to the doctor], by falling ill, yes, you learn by falling ill that there is a [certain] disease that exists' (13M 30–39 Swahili). To talk to other Africans about serious diseases was reported to be a 'taboo' (3F 30–39 French) and participants stated that the Internet and email were important resources for health information.

Explaining chronicity: imbalance and short-term treatment for symptoms

Some participants struggled to explain chronic diseases and there was sometimes resistance to questioning on the grounds that this information was specialist knowledge for doctors. Chronic disease was described as 'permanent disease' (18M 50–59 French) or an 'incurable disease' (16M 40–49 French). One participant offered an association with recurrence: 'a chronic disease is a disease which keeps coming back . . . it is like the flu and then everyone can have like me a cold, it is chronic' (17M 40–49 French).

At other times chronic conditions were described in terms of extremes or imbalances of normal physiological states. These diseases were often described as having abnormal states at each end of the spectrum. For blood pressure this appeared to be based on a layperson's description of the problem: 'hypertension it is when you have, your pressure is very high and hypotension is when your pressure is very, too low' (13M 30–39 French). For heart disease, however, one participant based their account on an awareness of medical terminology: 'you can have tachycardia or bradycardia . . . and if that goes up to 140 beats per minute the heart cannot cope, your heart is ill' (16M 40–49 French).

Diabetes was reported to be due to both a physiological and a dietary imbalance of sugar. This led to two ways in which this balance could be adjusted or maintained. First was dietary restriction and exercise:

> They say perhaps [you get diabetes] if you are eating a lot of sugar. I argue with my young boy here. He loves sugar. When he drinks tea he just puts in a lot of sugar. Me I [do] tell him. Perhaps the thing that is helping him is those [physical] exercises. (11F 40–49 Swahili)

Second was the use of insulin: 'it's like it's your sugar level and like constantly you have to inject yourself with insulin like trying to balance' (10M 18–24 English). Nevertheless, deep concern over insulin was identified by the only diabetic participant: 'I do not like medicines against diabetes: the injections every day! No, no I don't like that. I ask God to heal me' (6F 60–70 French).

There was also a belief that medication was only indicated for symptomatic – rather than long-term – disease: 'when we don't feel well [that is when] we take the medicines, if we feel well I don't think that the [medicines] will be important, even as a preventative' (17M 40–49 French). As a result hypertension was reported to require only a brief course of treatment:

> Interviewer: 'and if someone has got hypertension how long do you think they need to take medicine for?'
> Participant: 'I think maybe a week or something, a week, some, some may not need to take medicine, make to rest only ....' (15M 30–39 English)

Chronic disease as an acute phenomenon resulting from stress, exertion and older age

Cardiovascular conditions were commonly associated with stressful events and lifestyles, in particular resulting from hardship associated with seeking asylum. Heart disease was reported to occur in someone 'when he or she then gets to hear bad news or something shocking' (11F 40–49 Swahili), although one participant suggested a moral dimension by blaming envy of others' material 'lifestyle' as a cause of hypertension because 'humans are created with a heart of envy' (14F 30–39 Swahili).

Hypertension was perceived as a serious condition that could result in sudden, unexpected death: 'I think that it is a very serious problem, very serious. Because we have seen people die without even saying a word, straight away, because they have an attack of hypertension' (17M 40–49 French). Two people associated a hypertensive 'attack' with acute symptoms of breathlessness: 'Your breath is taken away from you and you do not breathe the air well' (11F 40–49 Swahili).

Two participants offered descriptions of disease in terms of sudden end points. One participant gave the following description of a heart attack: 'I would think it is a stoppage of how the heart pump the blood through the system you know ... dysfunctions' (15M 30–39 English). Another participant offered the following explanation of a stroke: 'it is like ... a crack in the nerves of the head, I think' (17M 40–49 French).

There was confusion for some over the role of physical exertion in hypertension. One participant associated hypertension with excess physical exercise, suggesting the following therapy: 'don't get yourself tiredness ... so you don't do very physical things' (15M 30–39 English). Conversely, another suggested that heart disease was more common in those 'who don't do that much physical activity ... like who don't do that much sport ... or who don't walk that much ...' (12M 30–39 English).

Chronic diseases were sometimes perceived as normal in older age. For example, hypertension was reported to be found in 'people in their fifties, it is not for young people' such that 'the people do not consider it like a disease, especially in Africa the people believe that it is a normal thing when they are old' (16M 40–49 French).

Heredity: an explanation for unexplained cases and an inevitable fate

It was striking that heredity was invoked to account for chronic disease when no other cause could be identified. For example, this was the only suggestion that one participant, whose friend died of liver cancer, could provide: 'I really don't even know [what causes cancer], well I think it is hereditary' (7M 20–25 English). Heredity was offered as a reason for conditions such as asthma, diabetes and obesity. At times it was linked to a genetic basis and even to an interaction between genes and environment. For example, one participant linked obesity to genetic predisposition and easy access to food in the Europe: 'their body already had the DNA ... because [obesity] was in the family and then, well, here, with all that they can eat here that can encourage the disease to come out [literally to "hatch"] in him' (18M 50–59 French).

In the absence of a family history, a related explanation of personal predisposition was employed to account for unexplained cases of chronic disease:

'I think that perhaps it is a bodily predisposition, it's like, er, people who easily fall sick from diabetes, and others, who do not fall sick from diabetes, and others who do not fall [ill], and I believe there is a bodily predisposition. The human body of an individual can be fragile and ready to receive that disease. Meanwhile the body of another person is not like that.... I believe that it is a problem of predisposition. (13M 30–39 French)

Family history of chronic disease was discussed as an almost inevitable fate:

for me here now I have already accepted that I am going in this family way, stroke is around in our family right now, and diabetes is in the family, here I feel it is heredity which is coming to me. (14F 30–39 Swahili)

This idea of chronic disease being a normal event within families was suggested by the language used by two male participants. One hypertensive participant stated that his 'familial' hypertension was 'not so bad' (19M 50–59 French) while an asthmatic man described his condition as a 'normal thing' (15M 30–39 English). Indeed, for one, acquiring chronic disease was discussed in terms of being a positive thing in the context of family history: 'They say that in their families in [Africa] there are some people have suffered from that [diabetes] ... yes ... yes ... also they have that ... and then they think that it is good for them because it is the family!' (18M 50–59 French).

A perception of inevitability was reported to motivate some participants to be tested: 'I used to be worried about diabetes because my dad has diabetes but I went to get checked and I was pretty okay' (7M 20–25 English). Conversely, it was reported that this belief led others to avoid screening: 'lots of women are saying 'breast cancer, ah no I have never tested [because it has] never happened in my family' (18M 50–59 French).

Accounting for perceived increased cancer in the West: unseen contamination with toxic agents

Contamination by chemicals in food was a commonly reported explanation of cancer and used to account for its perceived increased incidence in western countries. Chemical sources included unnatural fertilisers, chick feed for battery hens and preservatives or 'medicines' in tinned foods. Industrialisation in Europe was also implicated as waste was believed to emit toxins into the environment. Some participants offered their own accounts based on their observations of food production in Europe to support their view that food was contaminated with toxins. First was the different texture or taste of food: 'here you have the impression that chicken [meat] is soft, very soft, [whilst] an African chicken [is so tough] it can pull your tooth out... because this chicken has been running [about] everywhere' (13M 30–39 French and Swahili). Second was the greater size of livestock available in shops in Europe, in particular: 'strong fertilisers that help the fish to get big, to fatten the cattle, the pigs, so we say to ourselves "aha, here they eat anything." Even we are afraid because by changing [to this food] we are going to have cancer' (18M 50–59 French). Further evidence was offered in relation to the taste and strength of flavours in food: 'when you are cutting an onion your must cry, the tears must run, but here the tears hardly flow because [the onion] has lost its flavour' (18M 50–59 French).

Chemical contamination was particularly linked to cancer causation, with chemicals considered to affect the cells of the body. One participant described the effect of chemical contamination in terms of a small substance that changed the whole body: 'it is like taking a bottle of clean water, then take [some] colour and drop it into that water: it changes [and] that's the way the body is' (5F 50–59 Swahili and English). The effects of chemical contamination were considered silent and delayed, with chemical products transported throughout the body in the bloodstream. Indeed, one participant described contamination from chemicals in food in terms resembling metastasis: 'my body will just receive it inside there, you do not know if it will settle in the breasts, it will go to settle in the stomach, it will go to the legs' (14F 30–39 Swahili).

Not all participants offered explanations about where these beliefs originated from. However, one did suggest that doctors in Africa promoted an association of cancer with food contamination.

> since my childhood, well, the general theory that the doctors were giving in Africa at the time it was to avoid [food] stuff that was burned to excess and then, for example, certain [cooking] receptacles, to avoid certain cooking pots... which were giving out something that can cause cancer in the future. (17M 40–49 French)

Exposure to other toxic agents was cited as a cause of cancer. These included unseen waves from microwave ovens and regular use of a mobile phone. Finally, excessive sunlight and ultraviolet rays were also discussed as sources of cancer. In this regard one participant differed, suggesting: 'what causes skin cancer? I don't know, maybe some lack of sun' (12M 30–39 English).

Obesity, diet and physical exercise

Some participants volunteered that obesity was linked with chronic conditions, in particular hypertension, diabetes, heart attacks and 'problems with bones.' Only one participant linked obesity with more than two chronic condition: 'this obesity leads to lots of things and when the heart beats it tires itself and leads to lots of diseases like hypertension, all that, some little things like that and even the sugar level starts to rise' (17M 40–450 French). However, not all participants associated obesity with disease and some suggested that Africans were naturally prone to weight gain because: '[obesity] does not constitute a disease but it is a malformation...[because] Africans by nature are fat...I would say...above all the women naturally put on a lot of weight' (13M 30–39 French).

Africans were reported to be unaware of the relationship between obesity and health problems: 'obesity is a big problem but the people, they are not well informed about obesity' (19M 50–59 French). This was supported by one participant: 'what [health problems] can obesity bring? Well, I have no idea' (16M 40–49 French). This was despite it being such a problem that 'everyone has to change his wardrobe every six months because his size is increasing exponentially' (17M 40–50 French). One participant concluded that obesity was a consequence – rather than a cause – of diabetes: 'most of the diabetics that I often see they are a bit fat.... well, I do not know what this fatness is due to, perhaps it is the effects of the disease, yes it is that' (16M 40–49 French). At other times an association between diabetes and obesity was dismissed because 'somebody who suffers from diabetes can be normal [i.e., slim] like you and me. You will not know that this person has diabetes' (13M 30–39 French).

Availability of cheap food in the UK was offered as a possible reason for the development of obesity. Obesity was also reported to imply affluence – and even greater health status – amongst older Africans, although this was not necessarily the view of younger participants. However, traditional cooking methods were also held to be responsible. African food was at times considered to be unhealthy, for example using excess oil and lengthy preparation times:

> when you go into my mum's kitchen there is a lot of palm oil, like just a lot of oil, they are frying stuff.... when you come to eating vegetables we like cook them for a really long time and then add oil in them, so people when you eat well you might put on some weight I think. (10M 18–24 English)

One participant suggested that increased rates of cardiovascular disease amongst Asian people was because 'spices, I believe that they bring diseases like heart disease a lot... because a lot of spices are cooked with oil' (14F 30–39 Swahili). Salt intake was linked to heart disease by one participant: 'heart disease [results from] using a lot of salt at meal times' (11F 40–49 Swahili). Exercise was considered to be a problem for many Africans here: 'we do not do enough exercise, for example, most [Africans] are stuck in the house, that is to say are not moving, not doing much sport' (19M 50–59 French).

Discussion

This study suggests low awareness of chronic disease risk among African migrants living in the West of Scotland. Concern over infectious disease dominated participants' perceived health threats and chronic diseases were described by some as contagious. Overarching explanatory models were bodily/dietary imbalance, stress/exertion, heredity/predisposition and chemical contamination. These revealed some knowledge about chronic disease risk factors, for example, the relationship between lifestyle and developing cancer, between obesity and other chronic diagnoses and a role for the interaction of genes and environment in disease causation. Nevertheless, cancer was considered more common in Europe due to chemical contamination and cardiovascular disease described in terms of acute symptoms requiring short-term medication.

Our finding with respect to cardiovascular disease mirrors that of Beune's (2006) Dutch study, where some participants described cardiovascular disease in terms of acute symptoms and often associated with stress. Certain findings reported here are also common to studies of European populations, for example, perceiving cancer as incurable and implicating hereditary factors in its causation (Scanlon *et al.* 2006). Unlike research elsewhere showing that family history may not be recognised as a risk factor even by people with a large number of relatives with heart disease (Hunt *et al.* 2001), in the present study many participants were quick to volunteer increased personal risk based on family history. Nevertheless, at times familial conditions were perceived as less severe forms.

An interesting component of these narratives was the description by certain participants of chronic diseases as contagious. This perspective may provide insight into participants' understanding of the role for medication adherence and long term management in chronic conditions. Although anthropological studies show contagion theories to be important in Africa for infectious diseases (Green 1999) we have been unable to identify reports of such beliefs for chronic conditions. This perspective may reflect previous experience of infectious diseases in Africa. Alternatively, it may result from unfamiliarity with terms such as 'to acquire' amongst participants, most of whom were speaking in a second language. A third, important reason could underlie this belief: it is known that infections are indeed an important primary cause of many chronic diseases. This belief may, therefore, have arisen because of previous exposure to education about infective diseases in Africa, particularly concerning cancer risks associated with HIV. Other infective examples that occur in Africa include cancers of the liver, cervix and skin caused by viruses, chronic cardiac disease from syphilis and epilepsy from tapeworm infection of the brain. Knowledge that primary infective causes exist for common chronic diseases could pose a challenge to health promotion. In particular, this suggests a need to inform Africans about prevention of acquired chronic diseases through lifestyle change alongside existing interventions to promote knowledge of – and behavioural changes to prevent – infections such as HIV.

Participants in this study offered articulate and rational explanations for disease causation constructed from personal observation. Nevertheless, these findings suggest a need to inform Africans and promote discussion about their increased risk of certain chronic diseases. This was most striking in participants' perception that cancer rates in Europe were significantly higher than in Africa. This suggests an important need to challenge the notions both of cancer as a 'European' and random disease as well as informing African migrants of key risks such as prostatic cancer.

Explanatory models for perceived increased cancer rates in Europe were based on food contamination with toxins and this belief arose across age, gender and religious categories. This may also explain why some participants described cancer in terms of being 'caught.' Similar concern over canned food and fertilisers in cardiovascular causation has been reported from Ghana (Abanilla *et al.* 2011). These beliefs require additional research, not least because such fears may be real. There is good evidence for transmission from canned products of chemicals positively associated with cardiovascular disease and diabetes (Carwile *et al.* 2011). There are also case reports from Africa of fatal botulinum infection arising from canned food (Frean *et al.* 2004). In addition, we have identified Internet pages in Swahili linking canned and processed food to cancer. As participants in this study cited the Internet and email as important sources of health information, it is possible that the origins of these beliefs may lie in online or media sources. Alternatively, personal observation of decaying cans in Africa's warm climate could be the basis for contamination fears. These findings should inform health promotion in order to emphasise risk factor reduction through multiple dimensions of lifestyle change, rather than just the prevention of contamination. Nevertheless, such interventions should build upon the positive aspects of explanatory models identified in this study, for example a preference for preservative free and unprocessed food.

Additional implications for health promotion

Additional health beliefs identified in this study should inform health promotion. First is the notion that hypertension is a condition of older people and indeed a normal feature of aging. This could inform the development of patient-centred interventions to detect hypertension, particularly for younger, asymptomatic African migrants. Second is the perception that it may be inevitable for Africans to acquire chronic diseases already present in family members, although this was linked to a favourable view of screening and early detection. Third, there was the view that certain conditions only required medication for a short period of time, particularly when the condition is largely asymptomatic. Future research should focus on developing interventions to promote long-term compliance with medication for chronic disease, particularly in asymptomatic patients. Finally, these findings suggest a need to inform newly arrived African migrants of the risks associated from obesity, resulting from reduced exercise and easy access to high calorie food in the West.

Study limitations and strengths

In this study selection bias resulted from two factors. First, initial interviews arose from positive responses from certain churches and community organisations for Africans from specific countries or language groups. Second, use of a chain-sampling approach may have limited diversity in age, religion, gender and educational level. A further reason for few Muslims was that some participants came from countries where Islam is not widespread. The absence of male Muslim participants may have missed perspectives from members of a part of African society with distinct beliefs and practices (Rasmussen 2008). This is relevant to the implications of our findings because there is evidence that Muslim migrants' knowledge of chronic disease may be underestimated and because Islam may have an important role in supporting health promotion (Grace et al. 2008). A further limitation is that the relatively high educational level of participants in this study may have elicited explanations closer to Western models rather than private folk beliefs described in Africa such as taboo violation and magical causation of disease (Green 1999). The interpretation of findings is also limited by absence of a comparison group from the indigenous population. It is, therefore, not possible to draw conclusions about the impact of African origin and migration upon these results. The study would also have been strengthened by greater sample size to examine additional demographic character-istics, in particular socio-economic status, detailed educational level and age at migration. Whilst this was considered during the planning phase, it was decided that recruiting a participant group large enough to incorporate these variables (in addition to age, sex and religion) was beyond the scale and resources of the current project. Similarly, it would have been desirable to include UK-born Africans to explore longer-term effects of migration on chronic disease beliefs.

Furthermore, although the term 'Africans' is used here it is important to note that nearly all participants came from across Africa's central belt. Within African migrant populations there is known to be great diversity in diet, culture and psychosocial factors that impact on chronic disease risk (Okwuosa and Williams 2012). Additional diversity such as religious faith, language use and personal migration history can also influence perceptions of health and well-being. A further caution to generalisation of findings is that some participants belonged to small social networks and even within this reported a reluctance to discuss serious health problems with other Africans. A particular strength of this study was that it did not require interpreters, easing concerns about confidentiality and permitting participants to use preferred tongues. This facilitated participant recruitment and appears to have been important in eliciting accounts that represented wide diversity in nationality (albeit from Africa's central belt), cultural heritage and personal experience.

Conclusions

Like most qualitative research we have gained important knowledge about the perspectives of a range of participants and the agreement of our results with other similar studies implies that our findings include important overarching themes. Most notably these are the pre-eminence of infection in African migrants' perceptions of disease risk and a belief in increased cancer incidence in Europe due to chemical contamination.

This study contributes to the sparse literature of beliefs about chronic disease among African migrants' in the UK. These findings can inform education and training for health care professionals, for example, the importance of distinguishing with patients between terms such as chronic, terminal, incurable and recurrent. The findings reveal a need to improve chronic disease health literacy in Africans in Glasgow to promote their engagement with preventive behaviours. This should build on not only participants' existing knowledge of risk factors and disease, but also their self-reliance in the pursuit of a healthy lifestyle and desire to retain cultural knowledge and practice.

Key messages

- African migrants may have low awareness of chronic disease risk and, instead, consider infectious diseases to be the greatest threat to their health.
- Chronic diseases were sometimes described as contagious and explanatory models of their causation include bodily/dietary imbalance, stress/exertion, heredity/predisposition and food contamination.
- African migrants perceive cancer rates in Europe to be higher than in Africa and attribute this to unseen chemical contamination from 'unnatural' food production.
- Cardiovascular diseases were considered to result from stress Treatment constituted stress avoidance rather than long-term medication.

Acknowledgements

We thank the study participants and leaders of African community organizations for their involvement. Funding was received from the Scientific Foundation Board of the Royal College of General Practitioners.

References

Abanilla, P., et al., 2011. Cardiovascular disease prevention in Ghana: feasibility of a faith-based organizational approach. *Bull World Health Organ*, 89 (9), 648–656.

Agyemang, C. and Bhopal, R., 2003. Is the blood pressure of people from African origin adults in the UK higher or lower than that in European origin white people? A review of cross-sectional data. *Journal of Human Hypertension*, 17 (8), 523–534.

Aikins, A.A.-G., 2005. Healer shopping in Africa: new evidence from rural-urban qualitative study of Ghanaian diabetes experiences. *British Medical Journal*, 331 (7519), 737.

Aikins, A., Boynton, P., and Atanga, L., 2010. Developing effective chronic disease interventions in Africa: insights from Ghana and Cameroon. *Global Health*, 6 (6). doi: 10.1186/1744-8603-6-6.

Allotey, P., Riedpath, D., and Yasin, S., 2011. Rethinking health-care systems: a focus on chronicity. *The Lancet*, 377, 450–451.

Bache, R., et al., 2012. African and Black Caribbean origin cancer survivors: a qualitative study of the narratives of causes, coping and care experiences. *Ethnicity & Health*, 17 (1–2), 187–201.

Beune, E., et al., 2006. Under pressure: how Ghanaian, African-Surinamese and Dutch patients explain hypertension. *Journal of Human Hypertension*, 20, 946–955.

Carwile, J.L., et al., 2011. Canned soup consumption and urinary bisphenol A: a randomized crossover trial. *JAMA: The Journal of the American Medical Association*, 306 (20), 2218–2220.

Grace, C., et al., 2008. Prevention of type 2 diabetes in British Bangladeshis: qualitative study of community, religious, and professional perspectives. *British Medical Journal*, 337. doi: 10.1136/bmj.a1931.

Dalal, S., et al., 2011. Non-communicable diseases in sub-Saharan Africa: what we know now. *International Journal of Epidemiology*, 40 (4), 885–901.

Davey-Smith, G., et al., 2000. Epidemiological approaches to ethnicity and health. *Critical Public Health*, 10 (4), 375–408.

Dominguez, L., et al., 2009. Blood pressure and cardiovascular risk profiles of Africans who migrate to a Western country. *Ethnicity and Disease*, 18, 512–518.

Factor, R., Kawachi, I., and Williams, D.R., 2011. Understanding high-risk behavior among non-dominant minorities: a social resistance framework. *Social Science & Medicine*, 73 (9), 1292–1301.

Faugier, J. and Sargeant, M., 1997. Sampling hard to reach populations. *Journal of Advanced Nursing*, 26 (4), 790–797.

Frean, J., et al., 2004. Fatal type A botulism in South Africa, 2002. *Transactions of the Royal Society of Tropical Medicine and Hygiene*, 98 (5), 290–295.

Glaser, B. and Strauss, A., 1967. *The discovery of grounded theory: strategies for qualitative research*. Chicago: Aldine Publishing.

Graft Aikins, A., et al., 2010. Tackling Africa's chronic disease burden: from the local to the global. *Globalization and Health*, 6 (1), 5.

Green, E., 1999. *Indigenous theories of contagious disease*. Walnut Creek, CA: Altamira Press.

Harding, S., Rosato, M., and Teyhan, A., 2009. Trends in cancer mortality among migrants in England and Wales, 1979–2003. *European Journal of Cancer*, 45 (12), 2168–2179.

Harding, S., et al., 2008. All cause and cardiovascular mortality in African migrants living in Portugal: evidence of large social inequalities. *Journal of Cardiovascular Prevention and Rehabilitation*, 15 (6), 670–676.

Helman, C., 2007. *Culture, health and illness*. 5th ed. London: Hodder Arnold.

Helman, C.G., 1985. Communication in primary care: the role of patient and practitioner explanatory models. *Social Science & Medicine*, 20 (9), 923–931.

Home Office. 2010. *Control of immigration: statistics United Kingdom 2009.* Croydon: Home Office Statistics.

Hunt, K., Emslie, C., and Watt, G., 2001. Lay constructions of a family history of heart disease: potential for misunderstandings in the clinical encounter? *The Lancet,* 357 (9263), 1168–1171.

Information Centre about Asylum and Refugees. 2009. *ICAR statistics paper 1 key statistics about asylum seeker applications in the UK December 2009 update.* London: Information Centre about Asylum and Refugees.

Kheirandish, P. and Chinegwundoh, F., 2011. Ethnic differences in prostate cancer. *British Journal of Cancer,* 105 (4), 481–485.

Kleinman, A., 1988. *The illness narratives: suffering, healing & the human condition.* New York: Basic books.

Kleinman, A. and Benson, P., 2006. Anthropology in the clinic: the problem of cultural competency and how to fix it. *PLoS Medicine,* 3 (10), e294.

Krieger, N., 2000. Discrimination and health. *In:* L. Berkman and I. Kawachi, eds. *Social epidemiology.* Oxford: Oxford University Press, 36–75.

Levitt, N.S., 2008. Diabetes in Africa: epidemiology, management and healthcare challenges. *Heart,* 94 (11), 1376–1382.

Mensah, G.A., 2008. Ischaemic heart disease in Africa. *Heart,* 94 (7), 836–843.

Mullen, K., *et al.,* 2007. Exploring issues related to attitudes towards dental care among second-generation ethnic groups. *Diversity in Health and Social Care,* 4 (2), 91–99.

O'Donnell, C., *et al.,* 2007. "They think we're ok and we know we're not": a qualitative study of asylum seekers' access, knowledge and views to health care in the UK. *BMC Health Services Research,* 7 (75). doi:10.1186/1472-6963-7-75

O'Donnell, C., *et al.,* 2008. Asylum seekers' expectations of and trust in general practice: a qualitative study. *British Journal of General Practice,* 58, 870–876.

Office for National Statistics. 2011. *Population estimates by ethnic group 2002–2009.* Newport (Wales): The Office for National Statistics.

Okwuosa, T. and Williams, K. 2012. Cardiovascular health in Africans living in the United States. *Current Cardiovascular Risk Reports,* 6 (3), 219–228.

Parkin, D.M., *et al.,* 2008. Part I: cancer in indigenous Africans: burden, distribution, and trends. *The Lancet Oncology,* 9 (7), 683–692.

Pavlish, C.L., Noor, S., and Brandt, J., 2010. Somali immigrant women and the American health care system: discordant beliefs, divergent expectations, and silent worries. *Social Science & Medicine,* 71 (2), 353–361.

Rasmussen, S., 2008. Introduction – health knowledge and belief systems in Africa. *In:* T. Falola and M. Heaton, eds. *Health knowledge and belief sytems in Africa.* Carolina Durham, NC: Academic Press, 3–29.

Scandlyn, J., 2000. When AIDS became a chronic disease. *Western Journal of Medicine,* 172 (2), 130–133.

Scanlon, K., *et al.,* 2006. Potential barriers to prevention of cancers and to early cancer detection among Irish people living in Britain: a qualitative study. *Ethnicity & Health,* 11 (3), 325–341.

Vandenheede, H., *et al.,* 2012. Migrant mortality from diabetes mellitus across Europe: the importance of socio-economic change. *European Journal of Epidemiology,* 27 (2), 109–117.

World Health Organisation. 2005. *Preventing chronic disease: a vital investment.* Geneva: World Health Organisation.

Yach, D., *et al.,* 2004. The global burden of chronic diseases. *JAMA: The Journal of the American Medical Association,* 291 (21), 2616–2622.

Explanatory models of hypertension among Nigerian patients at a University Teaching Hospital

Kelly D. Taylor[a], Ayoade Adedokun[b], Olugbenga Awobusuyi[b], Peju Adeniran[c], Elochukwu Onyia[d] and Gbenga Ogedegbe[e]

[a]Global Health Sciences, Prevention Public Health Group, University of California San Francisco, San Francisco, CA, USA; [b]Lagos State University Teaching Hospital, Lagos, Nigeria; [c]DocSays Integrated Services, Lagos, Nigeria; [d]Federal Medical Centre, Lagos, Nigeria; [e]Center for Healthful Behavior Change, New York University School of Medicine, New York, NY, USA

Objective. To elicit the explanatory models (EM) of hypertension among patients in a hospital-based primary care practice in Nigeria.

Design. Semi-structured in-depth individual interviews and focus groups were conducted with 62 hypertensive patients. Interviews and focus groups were audiotaped and transcribed verbatim. Data analysis was guided by phenomenology and content analysis using qualitative research software ATLAS.ti 5.0.

Results. Patients expressed four categories of EM of hypertension: (1) perceptions of hypertension, (2) consequences, (3) effect on daily life, and (4) perception of treatment. Focus group discussions and individual interviews yielded a wide range of insights into the social and cultural factors influencing patients' beliefs and health behavior. Participants were aware of the risks of hypertension. There was disagreement between participants' own understanding of the serious nature of hypertension, the need for long-term treatment, and the desire to take long-term medication. Participants acknowledged the use of traditional medicine (e.g. teas and herbs) and healers. Different themes emerged for men versus women such that women often focused on family issues while men tended to discuss external stressors stemming from work as a cause of hypertension. Men were concerned with frequent urination, decreased libido, and erectile dysfunction.

Conclusion. Knowledge gained will inform development of patient-centered treatment plans and targeted behavioral and educational interventions.

1. Introduction

More than a fourth of the world's adult population (nearly one billion) had hypertension (HTN) in 2000, and this proportion will increase to nearly one-third (1.56 billion) by 2025, with economically developing countries bearing the largest burden of the illness (639 million compared to only 333 million in developed countries) (Kearney *et al.* 2005). Not only does HTN affect more people in economically developing than developed countries, but onset of cardiovascular disease (CVD) is also at an earlier age in developing countries (Pearson 1999). In two studies in southeastern Nigeria, prevalence rates of 32.8% in rural and semi-urban populations and 42.2% among a market population were reported (Ulasi, Ijoma, and Onodugo 2010; Ulasi *et al.* 2011). Blood pressure (BP) control in African populations is less than half of industrialized nations (only 5–10% compared to 20%; BP < 140/90 mmHg). These low rates of BP control may explain the relatively large burden of CVD in developing countries (BeLue *et al.* 2009). For example, in 1990, the proportion of deaths from CVD before age 70 years was 46.7% in economically developing countries compared with 26.5% in developed countries (Seedat 2000). Thus, there is a rather urgent need to develop interventions targeted at HTN control and subsequent reduction in CVD risks and mortality.

A major determinant of BP control is adequate medication adherence which is abysmally low. For example, in Gambia and Seychelles, only 26–27% of patients with HTN adhere to their antihypertensive medication regimen (Bovet *et al.* 2002; van der Sande *et al.* 2000). Several factors have been proposed as important predictors of medication adherence, but there is no data on the predictors of adherence to antihypertensive medications among patients in sub-Saharan Africa (SSA).

Considering that in many countries poorly controlled BP represents a serious economic burden, improving adherence could represent for them an important potential source of health and economic improvement, from the societal, institutional, and employers' point of view (WHO 2003).

There is increasing evidence that patient beliefs are important determinants of health outcomes (Beune *et al.* 2006). Specifically, explanatory models (EM) of illness refer to people's beliefs about the etiology of an illness, its course, the timing of symptoms, the meaning of sickness, its diagnosis, and methods of treatment (Kleinman, Eisenberg, and Good 1978). The provider and patient have EMs. A provider's EM is how practitioners understand and treat diseases and is often grounded in their medical training. A patient's EM is how they understand illnesses and how they choose and evaluate preventive or therapeutic recommendations and are rooted more in the experience of their social networks, their families, ethnicity, and culture (Fitzpatrick 1984; Helman 1989). Hence, health care providers and patients often possess different EMs of the etiology, onset, and progression of a given disease. Concordance between the EMs of patients and their providers has been shown to positively impact on patient outcomes (Weiss 1997). Discordant views may result in misunderstandings, conflict, poor adherence to medical recommendations, or other negative outcomes.

Researchers have used common-sense models and illness representations (Hekler *et al.* 2008), concepts similar to Kleinman's explanatory models (1977), to explore patient's beliefs about HTN and medication adherence. However, little is known about whether African and particularly Nigerian patients' explanatory models of HTN are different from what has been found in previous research. No studies have applied Kleinman's explanatory model or related models to Nigerians. Studies that have used these models demonstrated that the patients had explanatory models of HTN that differ from the traditional biomedical model (Beune *et al.* 2006; Blumhagen 1980; Boutin-Foster *et al.* 2007; Heurtin-Roberts and Reisin 1992). Studies of ethnic minorities have found that people belonging to different cultural groups (i.e. those sharing a similar set of values, beliefs, norms, and traditions) differ in their cultural views of HTN. This was found in a study of HTN between African-Americans and those of European decent where differences, particularly regarding knowledge, attitudes, and expectations regarding consequences of HTN (Snow 1983). This study is an important first step in illuminating the EM in this African population.

The objective of this study was to elicit the explanatory models of HTN among patients followed in a hospital-based primary care practice in Nigeria. Specifically, patients' beliefs regarding the meaning, causes, symptoms, and treatment of HTN were elicited. This study fills a gap by generating knowledge that can aid the development of culturally appropriate treatment plans and behavioral and educational interventions targeted at developing countries.

2. Methods

2.1. Study setting and participants

Semi-structured in-depth individual interviews and focus groups addressing explanatory models of HTN were conducted with eligible patients, who were recruited from the Lagos State University Teaching Hospital medical outpatient department – the primary care and general medicine practice of the hospital. The department is located in the center of the hospital for easy access to patients. Among its staff were 13 consultants (attending physicians) including the head of department, and several house staff/medical residents. This hospital-based practice serves most patients who need primary care service in the Ikeja metropolis and in 2003 alone, over 250,000 visits were made by patients from all over the region and representing a wide range of socioeconomic status. All individual interviews and focus groups were conducted on site. Patients were recruited between August and September 2006. Purposive sampling techniques were used to recruit patients who met the following eligibility criteria: age ≥ 18 years, diagnosis of uncontrolled HTN as defined as blood pressure $\geq 140/90$ mmHg or taking at least one antihypertensive medication, and fluency in English as English is the official language of Nigeria and the study proposal required that participants be able to provide consent in English.

2.2. Data collection

Potentially eligible patients were identified via chart reviews and referrals from their physicians. Interviews were conducted by a trained interviewer (KT) experienced in qualitative research methods, along with the assistance of several research assistants (RA). All interviews were conducted in English; however, bilingual research assistants aided in interpreting any colloquialisms during the interviews and focus groups. Individual interviews lasted between 30 and 45 minutes and focus groups between 45 and 90 minutes. The standard interview protocol composed of nine questions was adapted from Kleinman and Weiss' Explanatory Model Interview Catalogue (Weiss 1997). The interviews were introduced as follows:

> While doctors have special ways of understanding illness, people like you also have their own ideas, which may be different from what doctors think. It will help us to help people with HTN by understanding how it has affected you, what it means to you, and what you do to get help for it.

Patients were then asked the following series of nine open-ended questions:

(1) What do you call your illness?
(2) When did you first notice this illness?

(3) What does this illness do to you? How does it affect your body?

(4) What do you fear most about this illness?

(5) Do you think this is a serious illness?

(6) People explain their illnesses in many different ways, sometimes ways that are different from what their doctors think. What do you think has caused this illness?

(7) What are the major problems this illness has caused you? Personally, in your home and at work?

(8) What treatment is available for this illness?

(9) What kind of treatment do you think you should receive? What are the most important results you expect from the treatment?

Probes were used as needed to increase the richness and depth of responses, and give cues to the interviewee about the level of response that is desired (Patton 2002).

Three BP readings using the BpTRU device (VSM MedTech Ltd, Vancouver, Canada) were taken prior to the interview or focus group using a validated automated blood pressure monitor and following standard guidelines. BpTRU device is an oscillometric monitor, which can take a series of readings while the patient is seated quietly, and then prints them out or downloads them into a computer. The device takes an initial reading while the clinician is present, and then with the patient alone in the room, proceeds to take five more measurements at intervals of 1–5 minutes and then provides an average of these five readings. Baseline blood pressure was taken as the average of three blood pressure readings. Informed consent was obtained before each interview and focus group. All interviews and focus groups were audiotaped. Patients were given a monetary token for their time to participate in the study. Interview procedures were approved by the IRB of Columbia University School of Medicine and Lagos State University Teaching Hospital.

2.3. Data analysis

Participants were interviewed via individual interviews and focus groups until information reached saturation (i.e. redundant). This was determined through ongoing data analysis. The rationale and integration of focus group and individual interview data made three main contributions: a productive iterative process whereby an initial model of the phenomenon guided the exploration of individual accounts and successive individual data further enriched the conceptualization of the phenomenon; identification of the individual and contextual circumstances surrounding the phenomenon, which added to the interpretation of the structure of the phenomenon; and convergence of the central characteristics of the phenomenon across focus groups and individual interviews, which enhanced trustworthiness of findings (Lambert and Loiselle 2008). Interviews and focus groups were transcribed verbatim and content analyzed using ethnographic analytic procedures described by Kirk and Miller (1990). Content analysis was used to reduce the text into key content or thematic categories with similar meaning (Patton 2002). Both a priori and emerging themes and domains were identified that succinctly summarized the responses to the nine questions. Transcripts were analyzed: (1) pooled focus groups and individual interviews and (2) pooled by gender. ATLAS.ti 5.0 (2004) software for qualitative data was used to analyze the transcripts.

The method of phenomenology was used to generate domains of illness representations of HTN. This has been shown to be a highly reliable method when seeking to understand and elicit meaning of a given phenomenon, in this case HTN. Text was further catalogued by descriptive codes based upon themes. Text was annotated by, for example, illness representation 'cause', subheading, 'thinking or thinking too much.' Data were arranged according to themes, maintaining a reference to their original interview or focus group transcript using codes and primary documents in ATLAS.ti. For example, all participants who identified 'thinking too much' were grouped. Text was examined line by line, underlining phrases, and assigning tentative category labels and finally grouped. Methods for examining trustworthiness were based on Lincoln and Guba (Lincoln and Guba 1985). Member checking was accomplished by clarification during the interviews by the locally trained researchers. During the interviews, the researchers summarized the information and discussed it with the participant to confirm accuracy. Credibility was established by using the research team as peer debriefers. Members of the team not involved with the analysis as well as one external researcher not involved with the study reviewed the transcripts, methodology, and analysis to confirm validity and provide feedback. Confirmability and dependability were addressed by the use of an audit trail which included transcripts, a record of coding from ATLAS.ti, and notes taken by the interview team following the interviews and focus groups. The initial round of thematic coding was done by one interviewer. The principle investigator coded transcripts as well and the two compared results and came to consensus on themes. Examples of quotations are reported to exemplify and substantiate interpretations. Quotes are labeled according to the ATLAS.ti primary document number (P#), line number, interview (I) or focus group (FG), and gender (f = female, m = male), for example (P2:018:I:f).

3. Results

3.1. Participant characteristics

A total of 70 patients participated in the study including 20 semi-structured in-depth individual interviews and 6 focus groups of 6–8 participants. Eight interviews were discarded due to poor quality of information and corrupted audiotapes resulting in a final sample of 62 participants (12 individual interviews and 50 focus group participants). Focus group and individual interview data are reported together. Participant characteristics are shown in Table 1. There were more women than men and most participants reported their ethnicity as Yoruba (72.6%). On average, men were older than women with an average age of women of 53 years and men 59 years. The participants were educationally diverse with most having an elementary (primary) education (33.9%). Most participants were married and employed. An overwhelming majority paid for their medical care (88.7%) with their own money and had an uncontrolled blood pressure (71%).

3.2. Explanatory models of HTN

When asked to describe their illness, patients were generally able to accurately describe it as HTN, high blood pressure, or high BP. Their understanding of the

Table 1. Characteristics of participants $(N = 62)$.

	N (%)
Gender (% male)	25 (41)
Age (average)	
Men	59.4
Women	53.0
Religion	
Christian	48 (77.4)
Islamic	13 (21.0)
Ethnicity	
Ibo	9 (14.5)
Yoruba	45 (72.6)
Other	7 (11.2)
Education	
Primary	21 (33.9)
Secondary	13 (20.9)
Associate degree	12 (19.4)
College or graduate education	13 (20.9)
Marital status	
Married	46 (63.9)
Widowed	11 (15.9)
Separated	1 (1.4)
Single/never married	3 (4.2)
Employed	
Yes	37 (59.7)
No	24 (38.7)
Housing (rent vs. own)	
Rent	29 (46.8)
Own	29 (46.8)
How do you pay for medical care	
Others	6 (9.7)
Self	55 (88.7)
Blood pressure	
Controlled	27.4
Uncontrolled	71.0

terms was synonymous. The variability in meaning was noted in their understanding of the severity of their illness as indicated in the quotes below:

All I know is that doctor told me that I have been...that my eh...BP is high...I still believe that it is my BP is still high, but I don't know if whether it has run to hypertension. (P8:210:I:f)

...the only difference I could think of is probably, it's a little more serious than blood pressure, but it's a graduation of blood pressure. (P30:011:I:m)

I think high blood pressure is higher than...because it's when it has been established, you may be hypertensive but it's not ongoing. Your BP is not going up, but high blood pressure, you are already in it...(P4:033:I:f)

Although the patients described the name of their illness uniformly as HTN, high blood pressure, or high BP, the use of lay terms versus medical jargons varied as illustrated by the following quote:

> Eh ... it's high blood pressure but eh ... eh ... medical term for it is hypertension as I understand. (P37:019:FG:m)

They seem to think that high blood pressure and HTN are separate constructs as indicated in the quote below:

> Yes, high, high blood em ... pressure is ... is BP ... Ehn hypertension is ... the thinking. (P9:023;031:I:f)

In response to the question: 'When did you first notice this illness?' patients described being first diagnosed with HTN after being taken to the hospital for symptoms of dizziness, weakness, or headache.

> I was having dizziness; I was in fact, no strength ... nothing. In fact, I don't know, I don't know ... so when they checked my BP, it was high, very high ... so they gave me some drugs to knock it down ... so that is when I first noticed that. (P4:151:I:f)

The analysis yielded the following four overarching explanatory models as shown in Table 2: (1) perceptions of HTN, (2) consequences, (3) effect on daily life, and

Table 2. Taxonomy of patients' descriptions of hypertension (HTN).

Explanatory model	Subcategories	Concepts
Perceptions of hypertension	Thinking (too much) Environmentally mediated Behaviorally mediated Management vs. cure	HTN is brought on by stress or rumination HTN is a result of environmental factors HTN is a result of lifestyle choices, e.g. poor diet It is unclear if hypertension can be managed or cured and God is a determining factor in that outcome
Consequences	Death Comorbid health conditions Symptoms	HTN causes death or results in conditions that can cause death HTN causes other serious health conditions Certain symptoms may indicate that you have hypertension and/or that blood pressure is elevated
Effect on daily life	Limitations Medication	HTN is a condition that results in lifestyle modifications and/or restrictions Medication for hypertension creates problems for adherence due to cost, side effects, availability and personal issues
Perception of treatment	Medication Medical decision-making	HTN can be treated by a combination of orthodox and traditional medicines Doctors are experts and know what is best for my treatment

(4) perception of treatment. The taxonomy used here is similar to that in a study by Boutin-Foster *et al.* (2007) among hypertensive African-Americans.

3.2.1. Perceptions of hypertension

Perceptions of hypertension were summarized by four subcategories including stress-related issues and what patients colloquially termed as 'thinking' or 'thinking too much', environmentally mediated, behaviorally mediated, and issues of management versus cure. The concept of 'thinking' or 'thinking too much' encompassed ideas such as frustration and rumination about life issues and was one of the most prominent responses endorsed by patients as a cause of HTN in Nigeria.

> Yeah, thinking, if, if, if your brain is too loaded, with so many things, thinking of it, it can cause it [HTN]. (P7:180:I:f)

Environmentally mediated issues included circumstances that patients attributed to life in Nigeria such as poverty.

> I quite know that environment in Nigeria does not make it possible for somebody to ... of eh...our...somebody of our age to have normal pressure. (P37:216:FG:m)

> environment...the environment you live in can cause...even with...you know... ok...You know...in Nigeria...(inaudible) of the population are poor people, as in ehmmm...now that alone...can cause hypertension...ehen ..., and maybe...if you are in school, you don't have so many things and stress...(inaudible) tension...but then I was not in school, I was at home with my parents, so that was what surprised me...(P3:167:I:f)

> I think the biggest thing is eh...the...the social infrastructures that are not there. That we worry unnecessarily, which we ought not to. One of the...for example, let us take eh...this go-slow [traffic] as an example. You stay in a go-slow [traffic] for three hours doing nothing. And staying there alone will give you an anxiety and those social infrastructure that are lacking in our environment...(P37:706:FG:m)

Behaviorally mediated issues included lifestyle choices including diet, physical activity, and alcohol that lead to HTN. One patient responded:

> I just changed my lifestyle so I stopped drinking, I didn't...it didn't end with that I started jogging in parks doing many things to shed off my weight and when I came down, I haven't stopped. (P37:392:FG:m)

Uncertainty of whether HTN could be managed versus cured was prevalent in this sample. There is question as to whether patients were clear about the terms 'manage' and 'cure' because patients would state that it could be cured regardless of whether they take their medications. For example, when patients were asked whether HTN will return if they stopped taking their medications, they responded:

> No, it won't come back by the Grace of God. (P34:402:FG:f)

> Ah, Ah it can't come back again. (P9:198:I:f)

Some patients did state that they thought it could only be controlled and not cured as illustrated by the following quotes:

> I don't know if it can be cured, but I believe it can be controlled. Because I've never been told that it can be cured in an individual. I've always been told it can be suppressed or controlled. (P28:153:I:m)

> It's for the rest of life . . . I don't know what to say, usually many people stay with it, and I think its only control that we have . . . when doctors are giving you medicine, and you take it as you should take it . . . I don't think there is a cure; at least for now I don't think there is any cure. (P15:144:I:f)

Interestingly, the patients who confidently stated that it can be managed and not cured had received treatment for HTN abroad at some point. This could indicate that those who had exposure to treatment for HTN outside of Nigeria had been better informed about HTN by their providers.

Belief in God was central for this group of patients. Patient's believed that the outcome of their illness was in God's control as evidenced by the following quotes: In response to the question of whether it can be cured women in a focus group stated in unison:

> *by the grace of God.* (P34:348–349:FG:f)

Another example of the centrality of the role God played in the outcome of their illness:

> we use our medicine from the doctor, pray, and go. (P34:367:FG:f)

The etiology of the stressors was often different for women and men. Women tended to cite familial issues such as shock from death of a loved one whereas men more frequently cited external stressors stemming from work-related issues.

> I don't get hypertension before . . . one of my pickin [children] come die . . . so that's why. (P34:111:FG:f)

A gentleman stated his HTN began when his boss was arrested:

> he was arrested by the federal government, so I was . . . I was just met myself at the hospital . . . with a high blood pressure . . . that's how it started . . . (P18:059:I:m)

3.2.2. Consequences

Consequences were grouped into three subcategories, death, comorbid conditions, and symptoms. Many patients feared death or were concerned about death. Several referred to it as the 'silent killer'. Stroke or paralysis as a result of HTN was a serious worry for most patients. Diabetes was reported as a common comorbid condition and patients were concerned about treatment for diabetes.

> [HTN is serious] It is because it can lead to diabetes. (P33:125:FG:f)

Another patient stated:

> Emm-that hypertension I cannot explain much but I can explain on the diabetes. Eh, but what I know that eh...if somebody have eh diabetes he can have hypertension because they are working together. (P24:043:I:m)

Symptoms were a sign that patients had HTN and that blood pressure was elevated. Patients commonly cited pain in the body, particularly the chest, legs, and arms as signs of HTN. Patients frequently said that signs that their blood pressure was high were headache, dizziness, sleeplessness, and weakness. One patient stated:

> I'm having dizziness, pain...my one side of my body, both leg and my hands. (P25:032:I:m)

Gender-specific differences existed in the area of effects. When asked about the effects of HTN, men cited frequent urination and were concerned about erectile dysfunction and low libido or sexual desire.

> My fear is also that eh...it can cause stroke and eh...eh...at times...by extension, loss of libido...(P37:664:FG:m)

3.2.3. Effects on daily life

Patients discussed lifestyle changes that were necessary as a result of having HTN particularly around diet and moderate exercise, for example:

> he told ehnn his wife that she should not...she should prepare my food, separate...so she should not put maggi, and salt. (P38:262:I:f)

Patients wanted a cure so that they could go back to life as they had before HTN. Patients consistently responded that HTN has affected their mobility, inability to work, and negatively impacted their ability to earn money. This was described as a feeling of 'weakness' or not being 'strong' which kept them from their duties.

> Eh. due to it I have to...I have to leave my normal duty so that I will not be going far. So I have to find something doing nearby. (P25:231:I:m)

Patients stated that the effects of HTN resulted in limitations of their social activities:

> For sure you relationship with people will be affected because with hypertension you cannot be out going...You want me to come to a function in your house, because I am sick I cannot come. You put a call to me, say, oh I cannot come. Over time, relationship will drop and you find yourself just manning your house. (P37:752, 756:FG:m)

Patient barriers to taking medication included the prohibitive cost of medication, availability of drugs, and personal factors. Patients universally commented that medication was expensive and tradeoffs between buying drugs and food sometimes were a real choice:

Economical relief and seeing money to buy drugs, all the time to take. (P27:172:I:m)

The money to eat, I spend on drugs. Not even much money to eat again what you supposed to eat. Balanced diet...buying drugs. (P27:233:I:m)

It was not uncommon for patients to comment that they inconsistently took their medications. Patients stated that the availability of drugs in Nigeria was an issue:

It's not! In...in the pharmacy, they wrote me one medicine yesterday, I went to Juli (pharmacy) over there, because it has a name as a big pharmacy. (P15:199:I:f)

They don't get it...they don't have it! In Nigeria they don't have it. (P15:215:I:f)

Personal factors also inhibited adherence to medication regimens. The daily hassle of taking drugs was a factor for patients. These patient's responses well captured the array of issues patients had with adherence to medication:

First, I don't fear about it because with God, all things are possible. I don't fear about it. I know God can heal. I think you understand? I don't...I don't think am...much about it. But what I know is that eh...my drugs, I take it. When I get money I buy it and take it, not always oh. I don't take it every time. (P:11:089:I:f)

At times it's laziness oh. I think you understand? At times, I go feel this thing is too much, drugs every time. I don tire. 105 Ehm by the grace of God, I buy...I bo...I bought it as when the money comes in, but when there is no money, I left it until I get the money to buy it. (P11:109:I:f)

...I don't want to use drug all my life. So most of the time I don't take it. So it's when I notice that headache or that heartbeat, I will say maybe in the evening I will go and take drugs. So I don't like that aspect of it, they have not been able to find treatment. There is no sickness that I mean...I mean...., I don't know maybe it's spiritual, maybe one have to...you have to pray. You researchers or scientists or doctors, there should be a cure. (P17:086:I:m)

3.2.4. Perceptions of treatment

Patients perception of treatment was variable with regard to medication. Many patients felt that orthodox medicine was best and traditional medications could be beneficial. All patients reported that they would take the medication the doctor prescribed. Almost all reported that they heard of traditional treatments and many had tried traditional therapies. Several reported that more research should be conducted on traditional medicines. Responses regarding the uses of traditional medicine varied from patients never using traditional medicine, using it in conjunction with orthodox medicine, trying it and it did not work, and trying it and not certain if it worked. One patient reported:

...mix it together then we begin to drink, we call it Agbo in Yoruba area here. Yes... that means concoction...mixtures of some leaves, then all those things we mix it together. Then cook it, then we drink it. A times it work, a times when it a very hard thing, then we turn to the orthodox doctors. (P6:122, 126:I:f)

Another commented:

it can work, it can work...but I haven't attended to any of them. (P22:265:I:m)

Medical decision-making was an area where patients deferred involvement to their physician. Patients believed the doctor knew what was best for their care and appeared to lack the desire to be active participants in their health care decisions. Patients commonly made statements of that nature:

> Doctor can do what he wish for me, please…(P2:201:I:f). Whatever they gave to me, when I take it and it is good for me. I will start taking it. I don't know…I don't know drugs because I'm not a specialist on it. It's what you people give to us is what I'm going to take. When it work for me, ehen…I continue with it. (P13:389:I:f)

When asked what type of treatment she should receive:

> I can't say…I can't say all that…it's the doctor that will say: this is the type of the drug that you are going to take…because I'm not a doctor…(P7:281, 285:I:f)

4. Discussion

In this study, we elicited the explanatory models of HTN among patients followed in a hospital-based primary care practice in Nigeria. Patients expressed four major categories of explanatory models of HTN: (1) perceptions of HTN, (2) consequences, (3) effect on daily life, and (4) perception of treatment. Focus group discussions and interviews yielded a wide range of insights into the social and cultural factors influencing patients' beliefs and health behavior. An interesting finding was that although these participants exhibited an adequate knowledge about treatment and relevant risk factors as well as consequences of HTN, their awareness did not translate into consistently following treatment recommendations. Additionally, many patients considered issues of BP control to be the doctor's responsibility and placed a high degree of the outcome for their health in the hands of God. There was discordance between the understandings of the serious nature of HTN, the need for long-term treatment, and the desire to take long-term medication. Although participants clearly stated that HTN was a serious illness with deadly outcomes, they would also state that they did not consistently follow their doctors' recommendations including consistently taking medication. Participants rationalize (e.g. I feel fine) why they do not follow doctors' recommendations regarding their HTN despite knowing the consequences, known as cognitive dissonance. According to cognitive dissonance theory, individuals seek consistency among their cognitions (i.e. their beliefs, opinions). When there is inconsistency between attitudes and behaviors, dissonance occurs (Festinger 1957), and this was a common theme from participants in this study. Other studies have found similar instances of dissonance. In a study by Bane et al. (2007) it was reported that this dissonance was evident in patients between the chronic nature of HTN, the need for long-term treatment, and its asymptomatic presentation.

Overall, patients were clear that lifestyle, such as diet, alcohol, and exercise impacted outcomes related to HTN. There was agreement that medication and attention to diet and moderate exercise were important. Several referred to doctor recommendations and modifications they made as a result of being diagnosed with HTN. Participants acknowledged the use of traditional medicine (e.g. teas and herbs) and native doctors and healers. An interesting point is that although patients noted family history and some even endorsed heredity as a possible cause of HTN no one gave it a strong endorsement of its role in the development of HTN in them. In studies of explanatory models of African-American patients, heredity was a key factor (Boutin-Foster *et al.* 2007; Heurtin-Roberts and Reisin 1992). Even though ideas and perceptions about HTN were similar to African-American patients in the study by Boutin-Foster *et al.* (2007), the Nigerian patients attributed their HTN status to the degree and level of thinking rather than just the effects of stress or situational factors like poverty on the brain. Unlike other studies, the phrase 'thinking too much' is a very prevalent belief as a cause of HTN in Nigeria. We believe that this distinction is important because educational programs targeted at management of HTN in Nigeria should address this misperception.

An effect on daily life was the commonest area that related to medication adherence. Issues such as the prohibitive cost of medication and availability of drugs were common barriers to adherence. Many participants stated that medication was expensive and they often had to make tradeoffs between buying drugs and food. The daily hassles of taking drugs were also a real barrier.

There was variability across gender in the perceptions of HTN, especially with regards to patients' perceptions of stress and symptoms. Women often focused on family issues while men tended to discuss external stressors stemming from work. There was little variability in the knowledge of symptoms, but there were gender differences in the importance attributed to the stated symptoms. Men were concerned with frequent urination, decreased libido, and erectile dysfunction.

The strength of the qualitative methods used in this study is that it can directly elicit participants' perceptions, attitudes, and experiences. However, we are limited by the number of participants we can include and the diversity of the participants' backgrounds. Our study was limited to English-speaking Nigerian's living in a large metropolitan area who are patients of a teaching hospital and who volunteered to participate. Each of these factors is a potential source of bias and therefore caution should be exercised in generalizing the results.

5. Conclusion

Behavioral and cognitive models do not adequately account for the social and cultural variations in health behaviors. The strength of this methodology is that it can elicit an understanding of patient's views that are critical to improving sustained treatment adherence. Explanatory models of illness are significant for patient care for two reasons: (1) understanding patients' explanatory models of illness can lead to the development of culturally appropriate treatment plans addressing lifestyles, illness concerns, and patients' priorities in the context of their daily lives (McSweeney, Allan, and Mayo 1997). This may in turn help in motivating patients' adherence to medical recommendations (Garrity 1981) and; (2) Explanatory models of illness may shed light on patients' cultural beliefs with subsequent improvement in the doctor–patient communication and relationship, because discordance between patients and their physicians in belief systems may be the reason for poor communication (Betancourt, Carrillo, and Green 1999; Bokhour *et al.* 2012). An individual's explanatory models are subjective and personally created constructs of their environment, culture, and interpretations. These explanatory models are therefore potentially modifiable with exposure to new knowledge. Information from this study can be used to develop better patient-centered education materials that would address the misconceptions about HTN (e.g. it can be cured with traditional medicine) and its treatment. Easily accessible information on early detection, risk factors, and treatment is lacking. Health education directed at behavior change requires a thorough understanding of HTN beliefs and practices of the target population. To optimize treatment and self-management strategies, intervention efforts must be congruent with the individual's conceptualization of his/her illness.

Key messages

(1) Knowledge of impacts of HTN may not translate into consistently following treatment recommendations.
(2) Developing interventions that address the impact of HTN on daily life may increase medication adherence.
(3) To adequately control HTN it is important to develop patient-centered and socio-culturally appropriate interventions that will educate patients on the importance of controlling the disease.

Acknowledgments

This study was supported by funding from FIRCA grant 1R03TW0077452-01. The authors thank the moderators, recruiters, Dr. Tony Otekeiwebia, Dr. Thomas, Ms. Wura, the LASUTH nursing staff, and the participants and their families who supported this study.

References

ATLAS.ti. Version 5.0, 2004. [Computer software]. Berlin: Scientific Software Development.

Bane, C., C. M. Hughes, M. E. Cupples, and J. C. McElnay. 2007. "The Journey to Concordance for Patients with Hypertension: A Qualitative Study of in Primary Care." *Pharmacy World & Science* 29 (5): 534–540. doi:10.1007/s11096-007-9099-x.

BeLue, R., T. A. Okoror, J. Iwelunmor, K. D. Taylor, A. N. Degboe, C. Agyemang, and G. Ogedegbe. 2009. "An Overview of Cardiovascular Risk Factor Burden in Sub-Saharan African Countries: A Sociocultural Perspective." *Globalization and health* 5: 10. doi:10. 1186/1744-8603-5-10.

Betancourt, J. R., J. E. Carrillo, and A. R. Green. 1999. "Hypertension in Multicultural and Minority Populations: Linking Communication to Compliance." *Current Hypertension Reports* 1 (6): 482–488. doi:10.1007/BF03215777.

Beune, E. J., J. A. Haafkens, J. S. Schuster, and P. J. Bindels. 2006. "Under Pressure: How Ghanaian, African- Surinamese and Dutch Patients Explain Hypertension." *Journal of Human Hypertension* 20 (12): 946–955. doi:10.1038/sj.jhh.1002094.

Blumhagen, D. 1980. "Hyper-tension: A Folk Illness with a Medical Name." *Culture, medicine and psychiatry* 4 (3): 197–224. http://www.ncbi.nlm.nih.gov/pubmed/7408522.

Bokhour, B. G., E. S. Cohn, D. E. Cortés, J. L. Solomon, G. M. Fix, A. R. Elwy, N. Mueller, *et al.* 2012. "The Role of Patients' Explanatory Models adn Daily-Lived Experience in Hypertension Self-Management." *Journal of general internal medicine* 27 (12): 1626–1634. doi:10.1007/s11606-012-2141-2.

Boutin-Foster, C., G. Ogedegbe, J. E. Ravenell, L. Robbins, and M. E. Charleson. 2007. "Ascribing Meaning to Hypertension: A Qualitative Study Among African Americans with Uncontrolled Hypertension." *Ethnicity & disease* 17 (1): 29–34. http://www.ncbi.nlm.nih. gov/pubmed/17274206.

Bovet, P., M. Burnier, G. Madeleine, B. Waeber, and F. Paccaud. 2002. "Monitoring One-year Compliance to Antihypertension Medication in the Seychelles." *Bulletin of the world health organization* 80 (1): 33–39. http://www.ncbi.nlm.nih.gov/pubmed/11884971.

Festinger, L. A. 1957. *A Theory of Cognitive Dissonance*. Stanford: Stanford University Press.

Fitzpatrick, R. 1984. "Lay Concepts of Illness." In *The Experience of Illness*, edited by R. H. J. Fitzpatrick, S. Newman, G. Scambler, and J. Thompson, 11–31. London: Tavistock.

Garrity, T. F. 1981. "Medical Compliance and the Clinician-Patient Relationship: A Review." *Social science & medicine* 15 (3): 215–222. doi:10.1016/0271-5384(81)90016-8.

Hekler, E. B., J. Lambert, E. Leventhal, E. Jahn, and R. J. Contrada. 2008. "Commonsense Illness Beliefs, Adherence Behaviors, and Hypertension Control among African Americans." *Journal of Behavioral Medicine* 31 (5): 391–400. doi:10.1007/s10865-008-9165-4.

Helman, C. 1989. *Culture, Health and Illness*. Bristol: Wright.

Heurtin-Roberts, S., and E. Reisin. 1992. "The Relation of Culturally Influenced Lay Models of Hypertension to Compliance with Treatment." *American Journal of Hypertension* 5 (11): 787–792. http://www.ncbi.nlm.nih.gov/pubmed/1457078.

Kearney, P. M., M. Whelton, K. Reynolds, P. Muntner, P. K. Whelton, and J. He. 2005. "Global Burden of Hypertension: Analysis of Worldwide Data." *Lancet* 365 (9455): 217–223. http://www.ncbi.nlm.nih.gov/pubmed/15652604.

Kirk, J., and M. Miller. 1990. *Reliability and Validity in Qualitative Research*. Newbury Park, CA: Sage.

Kleinman, A. 1977. "Culture and Illness: A Question of Models." *Culture medicine & psychiatry* 1 (3): 229–231. http://www.ncbi.nlm.nih.gov/pubmed/617079.

Kleinman, A., L. Eisenberg, and B. Good. 1978. "Culture, Illness, and Care: Clinical Lessons from Anthropologic and Cross-cultural Research." *Annals of Internal Medicine* 66 (2): 251–258. http://www.ncbi.nlm.nih.gov/pubmed/626456.

Lambert, S. D., and C. G. Loiselle. 2008. "Combining Individual Interviews and Focus Groups to Enhance Data Richness." *Journal of Advanced Nursing* 62 (2): 228–237. doi:10.1111/j.1365-2648.2007.04559.x.

Lincoln, Y. S., and E. Guba. 1985. *Naturalistic Inquiry*. Newbury Park, CA: Sage.

McSweeney, J. C., J. D. Allan, and K. Mayo. 1997. "Exploring the Use of Explanatory Models in Nursing Research and Practice." *Journal of Nursing Scholarship* 29 (3): 243–248. doi:10.1111/j.1547-5069.1997.tb00992.x.

Patton, M. Q. 2002. *Qualitative Research and Evaluation*. 3rd ed. Thousand Oaks, CA: Sage.

Pearson, T. A. 1999. "Cardiovascular Disease in Developing Countries: Myths, Realities, and Opportunities." *Cardiovascular Drugs and Therapy* 13 (2): 95–104. doi:10.1023/A:1007727924276.

Seedat, Y. K. 2000. "Hypertension in Developing Nations in Sub-Saharan Africa." *Journal of Human Hypertension* 14 (10–11): 739–747. doi:10.1038/sj.jhh.1001059.

Snow, L. 1983. "Traditional Health Beliefs and Practices among Lower Class Black Americans." *Western Journal of Medicine* 139 (6): 820–828. http://www.ncbi.nlm.nih.gov/pmc/articles/PMC1011011/.

Ulasi, I. I., C. K. Ijoma, and O. D. Onodugo. 2010. "A Community-based Study of Hypertension and Cardio-metabolic Syndrome in Semi-urban and Rural Communities in Nigeria." *BMC Health Services Research* 10: article 71. doi:10.1186/1472-6963-10-71.

Ulasi, I. I., C. K. Ijoma, B. J. Onwubere, E. Arodiwe, O. Onodugo, and C. Okafor. 2011. "High Prevalence and Low Awareness of Hypertension in A Market Population in Enuga, Nigeria." *International Journal of Hypertension* 2011. doi:10.4061/2011/869675.

van der Sande, M. A., P. J. Milligan, O. A. Nyan, J. T. Rowley, W. A. Banya, S. M. Cessay, W. M. Dolmans, T. Thien, K. P. McAdam, and G. E. Walraven. 2000. "Blood Pressure Patterns and Cardiovascular Risk Factors in Rural and Urban Gambian Communities." *Journal of Human Hypertension* 14 (8): 489–496. doi:10.1038/sj.jhh.1001050.

Weiss, M. G. 1997. "Explanatory Model Interview Catalogue (EMIC): Framework for Comparative Study of Illness Experience." *Transcultural Psychiatry* 34: 235–263. doi:10.1177/136346159703400204.

WHO, 2003. *Adherence to Long-term Therapies: Evidence for Action*. Geneva, Switzerland: World Health Organization.

Coping and chronic psychosocial consequences of female genital mutilation in the Netherlands

Erick Vloeberghs[a], Anke van der Kwaak[b], Jeroen Knipscheer[c,d] and Maria van den Muijsenbergh[a,e]

[a]Research & Development Department, PHAROS – Knowledge and Advisory Centre on Refugees' and Migrants' Health, Utrecht, The Netherlands; [b]KIT Development, Policy & Practice, Royal Tropical Institute, Amsterdam, The Netherlands; [c]Department of Clinical and Health Psychology, Utrecht University, Utrecht, The Netherlands; [d]Arq Foundation, Psychotrauma Expert Group, Diemen, The Netherlands; [e]Department of Primary Care and Community Healthcare, Radboud University Medical Centre, Nijmegen, The Netherlands

Objective. The study presented in this article explored psychosocial and relational problems of African immigrant women in the Netherlands who underwent female genital mutilation/cutting (FGM/C), the causes they attribute to these problems – in particular, their opinions about the relationship between these problems and their circumcision – and the way they cope with these health complaints.

Design. This mixed-methods study used standardised questionnaires as well as in-depth interviews among a purposive sample of 66 women who had migrated from Somalia, Sudan, Eritrea, Ethiopia or Sierra Leone to the Netherlands. Data were collected by ethnically similar female interviewers; interviews were coded and analysed by two independent researchers.

Results. One in six respondents suffered from post-traumatic stress disorder (PTSD), and one-third reported symptoms related to depression or anxiety. The negative feelings caused by FGM/C became more prominent during childbirth or when suffering from physical problems. Migration to the Netherlands led to a shift in how women perceive FGM, making them more aware of the negative consequences of FGM. Many women felt ashamed to be examined by a physician and avoided visiting doctors who did not conceal their astonishment about the FGM.

Conclusion. FGM/C had a lifelong impact on the majority of the women participating in the study, causing chronic mental and psychosocial problems. Migration made women who underwent FGM/C more aware of their condition. Three types of women could be distinguished according to their coping style: the adaptives, the disempowered and the traumatised. Health care providers should become more aware of their problems and more sensitive in addressing them.

Introduction

Female genital mutilation/cutting (FGM/C) is a procedure involving cutting of the external genital organs, for which there is no medical necessity (Box 1: different types of FGM/C). FGM/C occurs in many communities in a large part of Africa. In

---

Box 1. Types of FGM/C.

Female genitalia can be cut in a number of different ways. Variations occur depending on which part of the genitalia is mutilated and the extent to which this is done. The World Health Organization distinguishes the following four types (WHO 2012a):

- *Type I*: Partial or total removal of the clitoris and/or the clitoral hood. This type is known as 'clitoridectomy.'
- *Type II*: Partial or total removal of the clitoris and the labia minora, with or without excision of the labia majora. This is also known as 'excision.'
- *Type III*: Narrowing of the vaginal orifice by cutting and closing the labia minora and/or the labia majora, with or without excision of the clitoris. This is also known as 'infibulation.'
- *Type IV*: All other harmful procedures to the female genitalia for non-medical purposes, such as pricking, piercing, incising, scraping and cauterization. Sometimes the word 'sunna' is used to refer to this type.

Somalia as many as 98% of women aged between 15 and 49 years are circumcised. FGM/C also occurs in Asia (Indonesia) and the Middle East (Kurdistan, Yemen) and recently also among groups of migrants in Australia, North America and Europe (WHO 2012b). The circumcision is usually carried out before the girl has reached puberty. Ages differ widely, with girls being circumcised soon afterbirth in Eritrea, whereas in Guinea-Conakry women may be circumcised just before marriage. There is a higher incidence among Muslims, but the custom itself is not Islamic. According to estimates by the World Health Organization (WHO 2012b), at present about 140 million women and girls worldwide have undergone circumcision. In Africa, some 3 million girls are at risk annually of being circumcised – which comes down to some 6000–8000 girls per day. In the Netherlands, some 60,000 women and girls originate in regions where FGM is common and are either at risk of being circumcised or have been circumcised (CBS 2010).

Female circumcision can cause serious physical health problems. Research by the WHO Study Group on Female Genital Mutilation and Obstetric Outcome (2006) found that women in Africa who had been circumcised experienced more complications during childbirth, including a larger incidence of Caesarean sections, haemorrhaging and a higher infant mortality rate. Chronic urinary complaints, cysts, ulcers, fistulas and infertility may develop later on (Almroth 2005; Morison et al. 2004).

In addition, long-lasting sexual problems are reported, including dyspareunia and vaginismus (Livermore, Monteiro and Rymer 2007), not only in infibulated women (Type III, whereby the vagina is stitched closed except for a small opening) but also in women with less severe cutting (Alsibiani and Rouzi 2008). Pain during intercourse is frequently mentioned and can have a negative impact on the relationship between men and women (Aydoğan and Cense 2003).

However, little is known about the psychosocial and relational consequences of FGM/C. While some research points to the fact that FGM/C may lead in the long term to trauma-related complaints, anxiety disorders, a distorted or negative self-image and feelings of incompleteness and distrust (Chibber, El-Saleh and El Harmi 2011; Lax 2000), a review of 17 studies into the psychological, social and sexual consequences of FGM concludes that the evidence is 'insufficient to draw conclusions' (Berg, Denison and Fretheim 2010, 3).

Most of these studies were carried out in countries with a high prevalence of FGM, but even less is known about the psychosocial and relational problems associated with FGM in circumcised migrant women in Western countries. The migration of large groups of African refugees to Europe and the USA introduced the phenomenon of FGM/C and its consequences to these countries.

Migration has its own dynamic, and the process of acculturation itself may cause stress and influence health and well-being (Berry 2008; Bhugra 2004). This migration-related stress is also responsible for the high prevalence of mental health problems among migrants (Carta et al. 2005), including depression (Vega, Kolody and Valle 2000) and post-traumatic stress responses (Silove et al. 2005). The prohibition of FGM/C in most Western countries may have a considerable impact on circumcised migrant women, since what was once regarded as normal, even indisputable, is now labelled deviant and repulsive (Johnsdotter 2007).

However, until recently only one qualitative study on the psychosocial and relational problems had been conducted in Europe, among Sudanese and Somali women in Manchester (Lockhart 1999). Three quarters of the respondents in this study mentioned recurrent intrusive memories and loss of impulse control. The type of circumcision, the associated physical complaints and the use of an anaesthetic were the determining factors for the development of a post-traumatic stress syndrome (Lockhart 2004). Overall there seemed to be a dearth of targeted research into this matter (Gruenbaum 2005; Obermeyer 2005; UNICEF 2005), even in the Netherlands, where the government has supported several FGM prevention projects within the migrant communities at risk of circumcision. This lack of knowledge was the main reason for our study. The problems faced by these victims needed to be more clearly identified for providers to be able to offer better health services. The study further aimed at generating empirically based conclusions about the impact of migration on long-term psychosocial consequences of FGM/C. As such the study is relevant to this special issue on chronicity.

Methodology

The study into the mental, psychosocial and relational problems of circumcised migrant women in the Netherlands was performed in 2008/2009 (Vloeberghs et al. 2011). Our research questions were: does FGM/C lead to mental, social and/or relational problems? And if so, what is the nature of these problems, and which factors contribute to the development of problems? Thirdly, what are the coping mechanisms these migrant women develop in relation to their problems and the above-mentioned factors?

Study design

A mixed-methods design was used (Creswell 2008) which is a highly appropriate method for difficult-to-reach populations (de Jong and van Ommeren 2002). We combined a quantitative approach, using culturally validated structured question-naires, with qualitative participatory methods, involving in-depth interviews with circumcised migrant women from different countries performed by peer researchers.

Using Grounded Theory, triangulation was sought in understanding the mental, social and relational consequences of FGM/C in a migration context, and how the women deal with those consequences. Hammersley and Atkinson use the term 'filling in the gaps' (1983), meaning that in the course of the investigation it *becomes* clear which elements are important and which are not. As such the understanding of the material and the answers to the questions develop step by step.

Study population

In the Netherlands, the largest relevant communities originate from Egypt, Eritrea, Ethiopia, Sierra Leone, Somalia and Sudan (CBS 2010). For this study, we used a purposive sampling strategy, including 66 women with variations in country of birth, age, marital status, education and type of circumcision (see Table 1).

Since access to the Egyptian immigrant women appeared to be impossible at the time, respondents were recruited from the other five countries only. A comparatively larger number of respondents (18 rather than 12) were recruited from Somalia and Sudan, as the most severe type of circumcision (infibulation, Type III) is practised in these countries, and the highest prevalence of psychosocial problems were expected. Respondents were recruited by the so-called 'snowball' method, which is effective in including marginal, hard-to-reach populations (Crescenzi et al. 2002). Snowball

Table 1. Socio-demographic characteristics of the research sample ($N = 66$).

Variable	M	SD	Range
Age	35.5	10.5	18–69
Age at circumcision	6.4	4.1	0.8–16
Years in the Netherlands	10.9	6.3	2–20
	N	%	
Country of birth			
Somalia	18	27	
Sierra Leone	12	18	
Sudan	18	27	
Eritrea	12	18	
Ethiopia	6	9	
Type of circumcision			
Clitoridectomy (Type I)	21	32	
Excision (Type II)	9	14	
Infibulation (Type III)	35	54	
Civil status			
Single, divorced, widowed	33	57	
Married with children	25	43	
Level of education			
No education/primary school	9	16	
Secondary school	24	43	
Higher education	23	41	
Source of income			
Job, social benefit	37	66	
No independent income	19	34	

sampling involves insiders in a particular group selecting individuals (based on certain characteristics) who are used to contact others who meet the same criteria. In this case, the interviewers approached women within their circle of friends and acquaintances, sometimes with the help of key people. The respondents were informed about the aim of the study by means of an information sheet (which was read out by the interviewer for illiterate respondents). Participants were reassured about confidentiality, asked to sign the Informed Consent form and told that they were not obliged to answer questions that they did not wish to answer.

To gain the women's trust and co-operation, it was important to actively involve the research population in the research process, both in terms of data collection and in interpreting and analysing data. Representatives of the communities were consulted on preferred terminology and phrasing of the questions and the acceptability of research instruments. Interviews were performed orally by seven peer researchers from the same country who had undergone circumcision themselves. These peer researchers were specifically recruited and trained for this study. The training provided by the research team concerned the aim of the study, the way in which the interviews should be conducted and how to handle possible risks and deal with ethical aspects concerning the process of collecting personal data. The interviewers met regularly to discuss extensively how questions were formulated, how answers were noted and how special situations were dealt with (such as respondents who refused to answer or did not understand certain questions). During these meetings they could share their experiences and reflect on possible effects of the interview process. Recruitment, coaching and monitoring of the interviewers were done in close co-operation with the Federation of Somali Associations in the Netherlands (FSAN) and other community women's organisations.

Instruments

The survey consisted of four questionnaires including:

- the *Harvard Trauma Questionnaire* (HTQ-30; Mollica et al. 1992), a 30-item transculturally validated screening instrument for post-traumatic stress disorder (PTSD) symptomatology (Cronbach's $\alpha = 0.96$ in the current sample);
- the *Hopkins Symptom Checklist* (HSCL-25; Mollica et al. 1996), which measures anxiety (10 items) and depression symptoms (15 items) and has proven to be useful as a screening instrument in several cross-cultural studies and patient studies (Hansson et al. 1994; Kleijn et al. 1998; Tinghog and Carstensen 2010) (Cronbach's $\alpha = 0.96$ for the total HSCL-25 score);
- the *COPE-Easy* (Carver, Scheier and Weintraub. 1989), which measures different coping styles by means of 32 items (Cronbach's α varying between 0.67 for avoidance behaviour and 0.91 for active problem-directed coping); and
- the *Lowlands Acculturation Scale* (LAS; Mooren et al. 2001), which assesses the level of cultural adaptation with 20 items and distinguishes between a global orientation towards the past (and land of origin) as opposed to the orientation towards the future (and country of current residence) in terms of integration skills and culture bound traditions (Cronbach's α for the subscales varies between 0.61 and 0.69).

All instruments were translated into the different languages, applying a back-translation procedure. A preliminary version of the questionnaires was pilot tested with 10 women, and both content and format were revised on the basis of the results.

Cultural validity of the questionnaires

For HTQ and HSCL excellent cross-cultural psychometric results have been reported (see Kleijn et al. 1998; Mollica et al. 1992). Reliability and validity of the LAS with different cultural groups are reported (see Knipscheer et al. 2009; Mooren et al. 2001). No data have been reported yet concerning the cross-cultural validity of COPE-Easy.

Semi-structured interview (topic list)

In addition to these structured questionnaires, semi-structured in-depth interviews were conducted with all respondents. The topic list used was developed in a gradual process using focus group discussions with peer researchers and local informants from the migrant communities involved. This resulted in a concept topic list that was adapted, amended and pretested during the training. The final topic list included questions about the circumcision itself, changes due to migration to the Netherlands, women's first sexual encounter, the impact of education and information about FGM/C, whether they have contact with non-circumcised women, and about their experiences with service providers in the Netherlands.

Data collection and analysis

The semi-structured interview was conducted during the first meeting with the respondents. Shortly (mostly one week) after, the questionnaires were administered. The interviews took place in the respondents' language of origin and at their homes. The duration of the interviews varied from 40 to 180 minutes. The semi-structured interviews were recorded and written down in Dutch by the peer researchers, sometimes with help from an official interpreter (with back-and-forth translation). Among all ethnic groups oral texts and the written transcriptions were checked by native speakers, showing little to no difference. The qualitative data were analysed using ATLAS.ti, a computer program used for the coding of qualitative data (labelling). The interviews were read and analysed separately by two researchers; important items were identified and coded. Afterwards the researchers' findings were compared and discussed with the research team to achieve mutual understanding and to reach conclusions.

The quantitative data for the five questionnaires were imported into SPSS (Statistical Package for the Social Sciences). All variables were summarised using standard descriptive statistics such as frequencies, means and standard deviations. Dichotomised variables were analysed with the χ^2 test or Fisher's exact test if any expected cell frequency was lower than 5.

Provided that the distributions were approximately normal or non-skewed (criteria < 0.5 $\alpha > 1.5$), mean scores on continuous variables were analysed with parametric methods using Student's t-tests for independent samples and one-way analyses of variance (ANOVAs).

The framework analysis developed and used included the different factors (e.g. socio-demographic characteristics, migration factors, health care in the Netherlands, coping), the way these factors are related to, respectively, the mental, social and relational consequences of FGM/C and the direction of the relations (reciprocal or unidirectional).

In line with the ethical standards of the research institutions involved, we formed a steering committee of external experts and appointed a doctor who could be approached at any time by respondents with questions or problems resulting from the research.

Results

The cutting experience

All respondents were asked about the type of FGM/C, at what age, who performed it and how they look at it now while living in the Netherlands. Most respondents from Somalia and Sudan were circumcised Type III, the infibulation, while most women from Sierra Leone and Eritrea had undergone Type I, the clitoridectomy. Younger respondents from Somalia and Sudan, however, underwent Type II, the excision, while none of the respondents remember undergoing Type IV, the *sunna*. For 25 (41.0%) of the subjects, the event was performed unexpectedly and without any preliminary explanation.

Table 2 shows the different demographic- and circumcision-related variables. Quantitative analyses show some interesting results with regard to these variables in relation to mental health. Women who were infibulated, women who remembered clearly the event of the circumcision and women who had had education concerning the circumcision reported more PTSD symptoms [$F(2.46) = 4.67$, $p < 0.05$ resp $F (2.56) = 14.48$, $p < 0.001$] and [$t(45.15) = 2.12$, $p < 0.05$] and more anxiety/depression [$F(2.51) = 4.37$, $p < 0.05$ resp $F(2.56)$ res $= 6.10$, $p < 0.001$] and [$t(48.22) = 2.37$, $p < 0.05$] than the other women. Women who were older at the

Table 2. Number, means and standard deviations of HTQ and HSCL scores.

Variables		N	HTQ		HSCL	
			M	SD	M	SD
Type of circumcision	Type I – clitoridectomy	20	42.65	11.59	34.50	7.59
	Type II – excision	8	51.14	16.38	43.75	17.81
	Type III – infibulation	26	59.00	21.41	47.19	17.30
Memory of event	Good	33	2.04	0.61	1.94	0.70
	Some	13	1.54	0.24	1.45	0.29
	Not at all	14	1.21	0.31	1.38	0.47
Source of income	Job	37	1.64	0.60	1.59	0.57
	No independent income	19	1.96	0.64	1.98	0.71
Discussed before event	No	25	1.57	0.57	1.59	0.62
	Yes	34	1.87	0.60	1.78	0.64
Education about event	Yes	28	1.93	0.71	1.90	0.69
	No	34	1.60	0.47	1.53	0.50

*$p < 0.05$.

time of the circumcision or with whom the circumcision was discussed before it happened reported more PTSD symptoms ($r_{ptsd} = 0.30$, $N = 60$, $p < 0.05$ resp ($t(57) = -1.94$, $p < 0.06$) but no more anxiety/depression. Women without independent sources of income reported more anxiety/depression compared to those with a job or social benefit, $t(30.37) = -2.09$, $p < 0.05$. When women were older when migrating to the Netherlands, they reported more complaints ($r_{ptsd} = 0.38$, $N = 63$, $p < 0.01$; $R_{anx/depres} = 0.37$, $N = 63$, $p < 0.01$).

Mental problems

But regardless of the association with these demographic- and FGM-related variables, respondents among all communities reported recurrent bad memories and nightmares at times, as well as pain, tension and fear or feelings of powerlessness and apathy. Anger, shame, guilt and feeling excluded were commonly mentioned emotions. Indeed, most women reported having long-lasting problems of some kind.

An indication for PTSD was present in almost one in six subjects ($n = 11$, 17.5%), as they had an HTQ scale score that exceeds the threshold value for PTSD. Almost a third ($n = 20$, 31.7%) showed an HSCL anxiety score above the threshold value, and one-third ($n = 22$, 34.9%) scored above the threshold value on the HSCL depression scale.

When asked what the mutilation meant to her, an unmarried 25-year-old woman from Sierra Leone who underwent FGM/C at the age of 12, answered:

> For some reason I became a frightened woman because of what they told me during my genital mutilation. They said 'you will be visited by a deceased person during your sleep.' They made it seem so real, I believed it. Since then I'm just scared all the time, and I cannot be home alone...This is all due to my circumcision. If a man makes a scary joke, it can get to me that hard it just ruins my whole day. Then I get really pissed off. Therefore, I say to my boyfriend that he may never surprise me or touch me from behind, nor should he address me secretly. And he does not dare make scary jokes with me.

Only one respondent claimed to be proud of being circumcised. An increased awareness about the health and legal consequences and many women's wish to prevent their daughters from misery and pain resulted in not having them mutilated when they were born in the Netherlands. The huge amount of media information – particularly since the Dutch government heightened its efforts to prevent FGM/C in the Netherlands in 2005 – awareness-raising campaigns and meetings among members of their own communities made the women more familiar with the consequences of FGM/C. Learning that it was not prescribed in the Quran, Hadith or Bible to genitally mutilate women fuelled the resistance of many of the respondents. They claimed that because FGM/C is related to culture, not to religion, it can and must be abolished. Media attention reinforced the conviction that they do not want the same to happen to their daughters. When asked how women around her had reacted when they had found out that FGM/C was not something that is done everywhere, a 34-year-old unmarried respondent from Eritrea with one son said:

> Women ask: 'why me, why us? We are all women. We all have the same organs, the same bodies, don't we?' Then when you start asking more questions, you find out why. And

the response is anger. Angry with your traditions, your culture and mindset. Until I came to live here, I had no objection to the circumcision of young females. If I had lived in Eritrea and had a daughter, I would have had her circumcised. But whilst living here, I have learned so much that I keep asking myself: 'why, why not other people as well?' Did they do this on purpose, and if so, why? I now realize that something was taken from me. That I am disabled. That's not a good feeling. Even when the pain has gone, there is the awareness. And that makes you angry with yourself.

Social and sexual relations

All but a few of the respondents said that they felt good about living in the Netherlands; they might feel homesick from time to time but overall felt safe and at home. Most respondents had regular contact with Dutch women. When the issue of FGM/C was brought up – some were asked at school, others when talking to the neighbours or to a colleague – feelings of being different, isolation and loneliness were reported frequently. Three out of 12 respondents from Sierra Leone replied to the question what FGM/C meant to them since they migrated that 'you start to isolate yourself' from people who have not been through it. A number of respondents felt that Dutch people they talked to about FGM felt sorry for them or pitied them. Accordingly, many respondents admitted to feeling ashamed. When asked why women who have been circumcised find this so difficult to talk about, a 47-year-old divorced Eritrean respondent with seven children reacted by saying:

> Because this is about feelings and more than that; it is about sex. You cannot share that with other people. You feel terribly embarrassed. That is why circumcised women become isolated, mentally ill or mad. Either that or she stops talking; she keeps her mouth firmly shut. And nobody understands why. It sounds shallow, but it goes really deep. The difference is that a woman who has been circumcised will blame any pain she feels on the circumcision. That is all we know. And because we feel ashamed, we stay home with our problems.

Migration to the Netherlands has not only led to a major shift in how the women regard FGM/C but to some also their own sexuality. Two respondents with children were reluctant to even have further sexual contact due to the pain it provokes and the demands of a lawful father. A 48-year-old respondent with two children who migrated from Sudan eight years ago answered the question about what influence FGM/C has on her as follows:

> FGM/C has a major influence on me. When I have guests at home I have to run to the toilet, which is really embarrassing... I never let my daughters be circumcised. I take care no one persuades them to have it done, and I will not leave them to choose.

> Interviewer: As for sex, do you think there is a difference between a circumcised and an uncircumcised woman?

> Yes, at least an uncircumcised woman has a normal life. A circumcised woman needs so much help. And eventually you never feel at ease.

> *Interviewer: How do you feel about uncircumcised woman?*

> I'm jealous of them; they are lucky. They have a normal life.

In a number of cases, together with the knowledge of being circumcised came suffering and anger. Migrating to the Netherlands had caused things to change with regard to sexuality. Some respondents said that a number of the men were now no longer satisfied with the women taking a passive approach to sex and were wanting their wives to act with a little bit less reserve. The women's partners had been influenced by the media and by the Internet – and in a number of cases also by having sex with women who had not been circumcised. A Sudanese respondent recounted how her husband would watch porn movies while having sex and would want her to try all sorts of positions: 'But I cannot possibly do what she is doing. I have been circumcised – she hasn't. So I will say to him, 'don't ask me to do the impossible.''

Some women were troubled by or even angry with men. Eight respondents reported feelings of despair, frustration and anger towards men in general, and their frequently self-centred behaviour in particular. In at least one case a divorce resulted from the inability of the infibulated woman to comply with her husband's sexual demands. Overall, however, there seemed to be acceptance of the changes due to migration and to the fact that men and women should be allies in bed.

General health and health providers

Women most frequently mentioned regularly having abdominal and menstruation-related complaints. Three respondents mentioned recurrent urinary tract infections ('every three to five months'). One respondent said that she was incontinent as a result of complications during childbirth and that she had been under treatment for 10 years.

Only three out of 66 respondents said that they had never visited a doctor in the Netherlands. Three respondents indicated that they were seeing or had been to a psychiatrist or ambulatory mental health provider.

When asked how they experienced health care in the Netherlands, many respondents answered that they often felt embarrassed, sad or guilty because of the way service providers behaved. The mere fact that the doctor saw their private parts during the physical examination and asked them questions was difficult for respondents. When asked why she did not discuss her circumcision with the doctor, a 32-year-old unmarried respondent from Sierra Leone with one daughter responded by saying that she was 'pigheaded.' She said doctors or service providers 'sometimes ask whether I have been circumcised, but I don't respond to that.'

When asked why she did not go and see a doctor about her complaints, a 35-year-old unmarried Somali woman with two children replied:

My family doctor is a man, and I don't feel like showing him my private parts. That means having to explain everything all over again, and that is something I absolutely don't feel like. I don't want to be reminded of the pain.

Interviewer: What does the pain do to you?

I start to tremble all over, and all the memories come flooding back. I cannot do anything for the next few days, and all I want to do is sleep.

During childbirth or when suffering from medical or mental problems, some respondents still felt reluctant to attend a health professional. Difficulties with speaking Dutch and an unwillingness to talk to non-family members about private matters (such as sexuality) are holding them back. However, previous bad experiences with health workers and their lack of knowledge about FGM/C were equally important. For a number of respondents the look of surprise or shock on the face of the person carrying out the examination was enough to make respondents blush or make them feel as if they had done something wrong. Being looked at in an invasive manner ('medical gaze') provoked a lot of shame. A 40-year-old married Sudanese respondent with four children of whom two were born in the Netherlands said about her first delivery in the Netherlands:

> Many health workers saw me during labour. They went outside to talk to each other, returned and then looked at me again. It took a long time. Finally I told them they should do a Caesarean section, but they said there was no reason for it. There were six or seven doctors in the delivery room with me. I was afraid for myself.

An Ethiopian respondent said that she thought her first visit to the doctor was terrible, and that she felt 'abnormal.' A 38-year-old married respondent from Somalia with three children said:

> You can see the facial expressions of the nurse, the doctor, the midwife. You can see their faces, the range of emotions and how they are looking at my body. That hurts...Those people's eyes make you feel sick.

Feelings of shame could reach the point where women did not seek help for their problems. But Dutch medical professionals who, in a careful way, show confidence in their actions and show sensitive behaviour and respect towards the women were able to smooth the tension and provide help. Overall two women spoke to the treatment provider about the psychosocial problems they were experiencing as a result of having been circumcised. Both said that they felt better after talking about it. One of them was an unmarried 26-year-old woman from Sierra Leone who had been circumcised at age 16. When asked with whom she discussed this, this mother of two children replied by saying:

> I do talk to my friend about it sometimes. She is a Dutch woman. And I also talk to a counsellor with the RIAGG [ambulatory mental health services] to alleviate the pain. That helped a little bit. Sometimes I have nightmares about what happened that evening. It still affects me to this day, but there is nothing I can do about it. Fortunately I am not in Africa anymore.

Coping with FGM/C

Respondents were asked what they did in case of problems or complaints. Respondents from Eritrea, Sierra Leone and Sudan often answered this question firmly and succinctly; however, most of the Somali and Ethiopian respondents were not very forthcoming. Somali respondents seemed to have more problems communicating about FGM/C. Talking causes harm according to some respondents. One Somali respondent put into words what in fact appeared to be the standard view among these women: 'I have to carry on with my life now and look ahead.' However, when asked what she did, when she was having a hard time, one respondent from this group, who was married with three children, replied that she would 'rather get into some form of physical exercise; that is more of a release. A lot of women watch TV or listen to music, but I find exercise more beneficial.'

Seven Somali respondents referred to religious activities as a means of achieving comfort and strength. Religion was also an important coping mechanism for women from other countries. Four respondents from Sierra Leone indicated that they would read the Bible whenever they were going through a bad patch. One respondent from this group said that she had forgiven her parents for having her circumcised: 'I would not have been able to do that without my faith.' Five of the Sudanese respondents and two of the Eritrean women sought comfort in prayer.

In the quantitative study, we found that a more avoidance-oriented coping style is correlated with the reporting of more PTSD symptoms and anxiety/depression ($r_{ptsd} = 0.42$, $N = 58$, $p < 0.001$; $r_{anx/depres} = 0.47$, $N = 60$, $p < 0.001$) and more substance abuse ($r_{ptsd} = 0.48$, $N = 52$, $p < 0.001$; $r_{anx/depres} = 0.58$, $N = 54$, $p < 0.001$).

Some respondents said they would talk when things were bothering them. In many cases, they would seek out friends or talk to them over the phone. When asked what she would do at difficult times, a Sudanese respondent (39-years-old, married with one daughter) who had been living in the Netherlands for more than 30 years replied:

> Because I came to the Netherlands reasonably young, and because I studied here, I have learned from Dutch people and through my training that I need to talk when something is bothering me. I talk about it to my husband, girlfriends and colleagues at work. I treat myself to a sauna or a jacuzzi or I do some exercise.

We expected the use of support-seeking coping to result in a decline in mental health complaints. However, a more support-seeking coping style is correlated with more anxiety/depression ($r_{anx/depres} = 0.32$, $N = 60$, $p < 0.05$), so women who sought support did not present fewer PTSD symptoms but in fact presented more complaints of anxiety or depression than women who did not seek support. The interviews showed that a number of respondents had indicated that they did not receive a lot of support from people who were important to them, such as their partners or mothers (in-law). A considerable number of respondents felt lonely and felt like a spectacle when seeking the help of service providers in the Netherlands, particularly when they were giving birth.

Discussion

Mental, psychosocial and relational effects as a result of FGM/C were found among all the respondents of this study. Symptoms of anxiety and depression were found among one-third of the respondents. One in every six respondents suffered from trauma-related symptoms. Respondents who underwent a milder form of FGM/C also reported post-traumatic symptoms. A combination of infibulation, vivid memory, migration at a later age, little education and language skills and inadequate support from the partner are concomitant with serious symptoms. In particular, women who were infibulated, who came to the Netherlands at a later age and do not hold a job indicated feeling depressed and anxious.

Migration to the Netherlands in many cases brought about more awareness, including about the possible health problems related to FGM/C. To most women migration appears to be liberation from the social pressure to comply with a harmful tradition, while at the same time some women seem to feel lost or experience a life of shame and pain. Confrontation with an environment that shows little understanding of FGM can result in feelings of shame and guilt. Problems with health care providers are common also in other Western countries: pregnant immigrant circumcised women in Sweden preferred to stay at home, even if they knew they had health problems, to avoid alleged insults from the midwives because they felt they were 'being stared at and being looked down on' (Berggren, Bergstrom and Edberg 2006, 54).

According to the 'mutual maintenance model' (Asmundson et al. 2002), pain may trigger the memory of what caused the pain, while this memory in turn may lead to experiencing the pain again. Migration and with it awareness about the consequences of FGM/C seem to trigger the recollection of the event and experience of pain. This coincides with previous findings indicating that circumcised women experience more pain after migrating to a Western country than prior to migration (Johansen 2002).

In general, it can be concluded that FGM/C is associated with chronic mental health problems, even many years after the event. Living with pain, particularly among infibulated women, appears to cause impediments and problems on the physical as well as mental and social levels. At the same time it became clear that serious mental health problems, such as PTSD and depression, are found among a relatively small sample.

When we discussed and compared our data, we started to see a taxonomy of different ways in which the individual immigrant woman copes. Apparently a combination of context conditions (such as relational aspects, the level of isolation and previous experiences with Dutch health care providers), combined with the perception of the cutting, the coping style of the women involved and whether she is capable of (self-)acceptance all influence the development of chronic mental problems associated with FGM/C.

The taxonomy implies a categorisation of groups of women based on how they dealt with having been circumcised and whether they sought help or avoided seeking help. We also looked at the degree of influence a woman said she felt she had over her situation: did she dare to say 'no'? Did she stand up for herself? The taxonomy identifies and points to some urgent aspects and in part implies options for service providers as to what can or cannot be addressed. This taxonomy was shared with the interviewers, who came from similar ethnic backgrounds as the respondents.

We distinguish three types of how circumcised women living as migrants in the Netherlands cope with the consequences of FGM/C: the adaptives, the disempowered and the traumatised.

The adaptives are overcoming the FGM experience. This group consists of women who are adapting, with different rates of success, and activists. The adaptives are troubled by problems (of a physical and sexual nature), but they are able to cope with these. They talk about what bothers them and, if needed, go and see a health provider. Some of them are in contact with their family in their country of origin, but in general they take an independent position. They might use religion as a key to adapt, as they know that it is not prescribed by any of the holy books. Among these adaptives are also religious women whose discourse about FGM/C (their reason for denouncing the present code of behaviour) had its roots in the Quran or the Bible. Religion determines their identity and the way they cope. In the case of Muslim women, the opinion of the *umma* (the religious community) is important. Sexuality is a private matter, and comfort and strength are found in prayer and in attending services. As a group, the religious women report less fear and depression than non-religious women, and this may have been reflected in their adaptive coping. This coincides with the findings of earlier research (for example, Brune et al. 2002; Khawaja et al. 2008). Religion may also give these women opportunities to relate to or become friends with other Muslim or Christian women (for example, Bos 2012). Then there are women who actively oppose circumcision within the Netherlands. Their agency but also activities such as walking, reading a book and talking about it gave them strength.

The disempowered feel angry and defeated; they bear their grief and do not see any way out. There are indications of substance abuse, eating qat or watching television endlessly. They do not talk about what was done to them; they feel ashamed, alone and disempowered. They either avoid sexual contact or dissociate during sex. This often contributes to the poor relationships they have with their husbands. However, they do not wish to divorce; they leave things to their husbands. These women behave in a manner which is inhibited emotionally, and they face trouble letting go of their negative experiences. Sometimes they have serious mental health problems but either feel inhibited or their husbands simply do not allow them to discuss these with a service provider. A tendency to fatalism can be found among these women.

The traumatised have mostly been infibulated and suffered a lot of pain and sadness. They are either divorced or have a bad relationship with their husbands. They are often troubled by recurrent memories, sleep problems and chronic stress (at the thought of having sex, when reproached by their husbands, etc.). They feel misunderstood by their immediate environment and sometimes by health providers as well. Women in this group consciously isolate themselves to avoid confrontation. Shame, anger and reproach (also aimed at their mother or mother-in-law) play a major role; however, these women do not know how to cope with these feelings. As a group, the traumatised report a significantly higher incidence of anxiety and depression than other groups, which illustrates the difficult situation in which they find themselves.

The broader picture

A circumcised woman leaving her country of origin and settling in a Western country has to cross a difficult bridge. Migration apparently triggers the momentum and speed of change. But change also takes place in the respective countries of origin. In most countries, FGM/C is now forbidden by law, projects are running and information is spread throughout many localities. Policy-makers, NGOs and media in Africa are promoting the eradication of FGM/C. According to COSPE and UNICEF (Landinfo 2008), families in Sudan and Somalia now choose the less severe type of FGM/C so as 'to protect their daughters from infibulation and in order to avoid that their daughters become victims of social stigmatisation.' With the long-lasting effects of the problems related to infibulation, this means healthy progress.

On the other hand, however, FGM/C appears to be a deep-rooted cultural practice. Even nowadays among many ethnic communities in Africa an uncircumcised woman still bears the risk of being considered an outcast (IPPF 2008). A study in Nigeria shows the difference in prevalence between Yoruba mothers and daughters only slightly lowered from 75% to 71%, even though 53% of the respondents are aware of the health hazards (Akinsanya 2011). Change will come step-by-step, rather than suddenly. Stigmatising the targeted women and cultures is, however, not a way forward. According to a UNICEF (2004) advocacy paper on FGM/C, 'rather than judging and condemning Somali society, a sensitive long-term approach is needed that takes into account the local context.' Regarding the topic of this article – the way women cope with the chronic consequences of FGM/C – our study shows the struggle of some respondents and their ineffective dealing with their complaints, but also that others learned to talk about their problems, broke the taboo and often find consolation, support and strength with each other. For the mothers the harm may already have been done, but many want to protect their daughters from enduring the same suffering. In some places in Africa a temporary transitional compromise is sought instead, and a less severe type of circumcision is done in hospitals or clinics and with the use of anaesthetics: the medicalization of FGM/C (e.g. Rasheed, Abd-Ellah and Yousef 2011). Whether that is a positive development remains an issue of debate. According to the WHO, even if health complications at the time of the operation diminish, the human right of the child is still breached, its physical integrity is damaged and the underlying subordinate position of women is untouched (Cook 2008). And at what cost? Instead: 'African health ministries that invest in curbing the practice of FGM are likely to recover a large portion of the investment by saving money from prevented obstetric complications... [and] of treating FGM-related psychological and sexual health problems' (Adam et al. 2010).

Methodological considerations

Although the results of this study support the claim that FGM/C exerts a major negative impact on mental health beyond somatic complications, some caution is warranted in interpreting these results.

The small group size presents an important limitation, and the results do not allow general conclusions about the prevalence of psychiatric disorders after FGM/C. The composition characteristics of the group (i.e. the low age and the high level of education) might also have an influence on the findings of this study. The attempt to interview women with lower education levels with a female interpreter did not work out because of the sensitive subject and the highly secretive nature of FGM/C.

We tried to enhance the reliability by seeking the same information in different questions. Ethnic matching of the interviewers may work out positively (people may be more open-hearted and more honest toward an ethnically similar interviewer, and this may contribute to a more contextualised and in-depth understanding of the challenges the women face) as well as negatively (it is harder talking honestly about taboo issues, also because of the fear of gossip, which may bias the data). Selection bias influencing the results seems a probability, as all respondents were willing to talk to the interviewers about their FGM/C and its effects. It is possible that women who do not want to talk about the issue and were not included in this study suffer more or other symptoms. There is also a chance that those women advocating for the practice were either not approached or were unwilling to be interviewed for fear it would cause them trouble (see Knipscheer & Kleber (2004a, 2004b) for similar findings concerning the effect of ethnic matching in dyads).

Notwithstanding the limitations, our study undoubtedly has a unique and innovative character. The way we recruited respondents, the active and motivated participation of the target population as well as the mixed-methods strategy through which we obtained our data provide sufficient grounds for answering the research questions validly.

Conclusions

A selection of data from our study in the Netherlands was used to show that FGM/C is associated with mental, psychosocial and relational problems for a considerable number of migrant women. Under certain circumstances, these problems may develop into a poor mental health condition of a chronic nature. Migration appears to be an influence, but also of great importance is the way in which the women cope with their new situation and how their intimates, health care providers and the people with whom they have contact react. The way the women cope with the migrant situation and the problems they have differ considerably. Health care providers should be alert to what cues may be indicative of chronic problems and enhance their (intercultural) communication skills in relation to these problems.

Key messages

(1) Migration influences the perception of the immigrant women of the consequences of FGM/C.
(2) In a number of cases migration to a Western country may result in chronic psychosocial and sexual problems.
(3) Attentive communication skills are required when providing care or cure.

Acknowledgements

The study was conducted with the financial support of a health insurance company (SASS) and the Foundation for Assistance to Victims (Slachtofferhulp).

References

Adam, T., H. Bathija, D. Bishai, Y. -T. Bonnenfant, M. Darwish, D. Huntington, and E. Johansen. 2010. "Estimating the Obstetric Cost of Female Genital Mutilation in Six African Countries." *Bulletin WHO* 88: 281–288. http://www.who.int/bulletin/volumes/88/4/09-064808.pdf.

Akinsanya, A. and G. Babatunde. 2011. "Intergenerational Attitude Change Regarding Female Genital Cutting in Yourba Speaking Ethnic Group of Southwest Nigeria: A Qualitative and Quantitative Enquiry." *Electronic Journal of Human Sexuality* 14. Accessed September 27, 2011. http://www.ejhs.org/volume14/FGC.htm

Almroth L. 2005. "Genital Mutilation of Girls in Sudan: Community- and Hospital-Based Studies on Female Genital Cutting and its Sequelae." Thesis. Stockholm: Karolinska Institute. Accessed September 28, 2011. http://diss.kib.ki.se/2005/91-7140-236-5/thesis.pdf

Alsibiani, S., and A. Rouzi. 2008. "Sexual Function in Women with Female Genital Mutilation." *Fertility & Sterility* 93 (3): 722–724. doi:10.1016/j.fertnstert.2008.10.035.

Asmundson, G., M. Coons, S. Taylor, and J. Katz. 2002. "PTSD and the Experience of Pain: Research and Clinical Implications of Shared Vulnerability and Mutual Maintenance Models." *Canadian Journal Psychiatry* 47 (10): 930–937.

Aydoğan, S., and M. Cense. 2003. *Reactie op Casus 8. Wankele waarden. Levenskwesties van moslims belicht door professionals* [Response to Case 8. Unstable Values. Life Issues Among Muslims Clarified by Professionals]. Utrecht: Forum.

Berg, R., E. Denison, and A. Fretheim. 2010. "Psychological, Social and Sexual Consequences of Female Genital Mutilation/Cutting (FGM/C): A Systematic Review of Quantitative Studies." Report from Kunnskapssenteret (Norway). Accessed April 11, 2011. http://www.kunnskapssenteret.no/publikasjoner/9555.cms?threepage=1

Berggren, V., S. Bergstrom, and A. -K. Edberg. 2006. "Being Different and Vulnerable: Experiences of Immigrant African Women Who Have Been Circumcised and Sought Maternal Care in Sweden." *Journal of Transcultural Nursing* 17 (1): 50–57. doi:10.1177/1043659605281981.

Berry, J. 2008. "Globalisation and Acculturation." *International Journal of Intercultural Relations* 32: 328–336. doi:10.1016/j.ijintrel.2008.04.001.

Bhugra, D. 2004. "Migration and Mental Health." *Acta Psychiatrica Scandinavica* 109: 243–258. doi:10.1046/j.0001-690X.2003.00246.x.

Bos, M. 2012. "Vrouw Zijn – Seksualiteit en seksuele beleving van Somalische vrouwen voor en na migratie [Being Woman – Sexuality and Sexual Experiences of Somali Women Before and After Migration]." Doctoral Thesis. Amsterdam: Universiteit van Amsterdam.

Brune, M., C. Haasen, M. Krausz, O. Yagdiran, E. Bustos, and D. Eisenman. 2002. "Belief Systems as Coping Factors for Traumatized Refugees: A Pilot Study." *European Psychiatry* 17: 451–458. doi:10.1016/S0924-9338(02)00708-3.

Carta, Mg., M. Bernal, Mg. Hardoy, and J. M. Haro-Abad. 2005. "Migration and Mental Health in Europe (The State of the Mental Health in Europe Working Group: Appendix 1)." *Clinical Practice Epidemiological Mental Health* 1: 13. doi:10.1186/1745-0179-1-13

Carver, C., M. Scheier, and J. Weintraub. 1989. "Assessing Coping Strategies: A Theoretically Base Approach." *Journal of Personality and Social Psychology* 57 (2): 267–283. doi:10.1037/0022-3514.56.2.267.

CBS. 2010. Centraal Bureau Statistieken-data. Den Haag. Accessed September 9, 2011. http://statline.cbs.nl/StatWeb

Chibber, R., E El-Saleh, and J. El Harmi. 2011. "Female Circumcision: Obstetrical and Psychological Sequelae Continues Unabated in the 21st century." *Journal of Maternal-Fetal and Neonatal Medicine* 24 (6): 833–836. doi:10.3109/14767058.2010.531318.

Cook, R. 2008. "Ethical concerns in female genital cutting." *African Journal of Reproductive Health* 12: 7–11. http://www.bioline.org.br/pdf?rh08001.

Crescenzi, A., E. Ketzer, M. van Ommeren, K. Phuntsok, I. Komproe, and J. de Jong. 2002. "Effect of Political Imprisonment and Trauma History on Recent Tibetan Refugees in India." *Journal of Traumatic Stress* 15 (5): 369–375. doi:10.1023/A:1020129107279.

Creswell, J. 2008. *Research Design: Qualitative, Quantitative and Mixed Methods Approaches.* 3rd ed. Thousand Oaks: Sage.

de Jong, J., and M. van Ommeren. 2002. "Toward A Culture-Informed Epidemiology: Combining Qualitative and Quantitative Research in Transcultural Contexts." *Transcult Psychiatry* 39 (4): 422–433. doi:10.1177/136346150203900402.

Gruenbaum, E. 2005. "Socio-Cultural Dynamics of Female Genital Cuttings: Research Findings, Gaps and Directions." *Culture, Health & Sexuality* 7 (5): 429–441. doi:10.1080/13691050500262953.

Hammersley, M., and P. Atkinson. 1983. *Ethnography: Principles in practice.* London: Tavistock.

Hansson, L., R. Nettelbladt, L. Borgquist, and G. Nordström. 1994. "Screening for psychiatric illness in primary care." *Social Psychiatry and Psychiatric Epidemiology* 29: 83–87.

International Planned Parenthood Federation (IPPF). 2008. Briefing paper Female genital mutilation. accessed December 21, 2012 http://www.ippf.org/resources/publications/ippf-briefing-paper-female-genital-mutilation

Johansen, R. 2002. "Pain as a Counterpoint to Culture. Analysis of Pain Associated With Infibulation Among Somali Immigrants in Norway." *Medical Anthropology Quarterly* 16 (3): 312–340. doi:10.1525/maq.2002.16.3.312.

Johnsdotter, S. 2007. "Persistence of Tradition or Reassessment of Cultural Practices in Exile? Discourses on Female Circumcision among and About Swedish Somalis." In *Transcultural Bodies. Female Genital Cutting in Global Context*, edited by Y. Hernlund and B. Shell-Duncan, 107–134. New Jersey, NJ: Rutgers University Press.

Khawaja, N., K. White, R. Schweitzer, and J. Greenslade. 2008. "Difficulties and Coping Strategies of Sudanese Refugees: A Qualitative Approach." *Transcultural Psychiatry* 45 (3): 489–512. doi:10.1177/1363461508094678.

Kleijn, W., J. Hovens, J. Rodenburg, and R. Rijnders. 1998. "Psychiatrische symptomen bij vluchtelingen aangemeld bij het psychiatrisch centrum De Vonk [Psychiatric Symptoms among 710 Refugees Registered at the Psychiatric Center De Vonk]." *Nederlands Tijdschrift voor Geneeskunde* 142 (30): 1724–1728.

Knipscheer, J. W., and R. J. Kleber. 2004a. "The Importance of Ethnic Similarity in the Therapist-Patient Dyad Among Surinamese Migrants in Dutch Mental Health Care." *Psychology and Psychotherapy: Theory, Research and Practice* 77: 273–278. doi:10.1348/147608304323112537.

Knipscheer, J. W., and R. J. Kleber. 2004b. "A Need for Ethnic Similarity in the Therapist-Patient Interaction? Mediterranean Migrants in Dutch Mental Health Care." *Journal of Clinical Psychology* 60 (6): 543–554. doi:10.1002/jclp.20008.

Knipscheer, J., A. Drogendijk, C. Gülsen, and R. Kleber. 2009. "Differences and Similarities in Posttraumatic stress Between Economic Migrants and Forced Migrants: Acculturation and Mental Health within a Turkish and a Kurdish Sample." *International Journal of Clinical and Health Psychology* 9 (3): 373–391.

Landinfo. 2008. Report Female Genital Mutilation in Sudan and Somalia. Oslo: Country of Origin Information Centre. Accessed September 15, 2011. http://www.landinfo.no/asset/764/1/764_1.pdf

Lax, R. 2000. "Socially Sanctioned Violence Against Women: Female Genital Mutilation Is Its Most Brutal Form." *Clinical Social Work Journal* 28 (4): 403–412. doi:10.1023/A:1005119906627.

Livermore, L., R. Monteiro, and J. Rymer. 2007. "Attitudes and Awareness of Female Genital Mutilation: A Questionnaire-Based Study in a Kenyan Hospital." *Journal of Obstetrics and Gynaecology* 27 (8): 816–818. doi:10.1080/01443610701709650.

Lockhart, H. 1999. *A Preliminary Investigation of the Psychological Effects of Female Circumcision (FGM)*. Unpublished Doctorate in Clinical Psychology, Faculty of Medicine. Manchester: University of Manchester.

Lockhart, H. 2004. *Female Genital Mutilation: Treating the Tears*. London: Middlesex University Press.

Mollica, R., Y. Caspin-Yavin, P. Bollini, T. Truong, S. Tor, and J. Lavelle. 1992. "The Harvard Trauma Questionnaire. Validating A Cross-Cultural Instrument for Measuring Torture, Trauma and Posttraumatic Stress Disorder in Indochinese Refugees." *The Journal of Nervous and Mental Disease* 180: 110–115. doi:10.1097/00005053-199202000-00008.

Mollica, R., G. Wyshak, T. de Marnette, B. Tu, T. Yang, F. Khuon, R. Coelho, and J. Lavelle. 1996. "*Hopkins Symptom Checklist (HSCL-25): Manual for Cambodian, Laotian and Vietnamese Versions.*" *Torture* 6: 35–42.

Mooren, T., J. Knipscheer, A. Kamperman, R. Kleber, and Komproe I. 2001. "The Lowlands Acculturation Scale: Validity of an Adaptation Measure among Migrants in The Netherlands." In *The Impact of War. Studies on the Psychological Consequences of War and Migration*, edited by T. Mooren, 44–68. Delft: Eburon.

Morison, L., A. Dirir, S. Elmi, J. Warsame, and S. Dirir. 2004. "How Experiences and Attitudes Relating to Female Circumcision Vary According to Age on Arrival in Britain: A Study Among Young Somalis in London." *Ethnicity and Health* 9: 75–100. doi:10.1080/1355785042000202763.

Obermeyer, C. 2005. "The Consequences of Female Circumcision for Health and Sexuality: An Update on the Evidence." *Culture, Health & Sexuality* 7 (5): 443–461. doi:10.1080/14789940500181495.

Rasheed, S., A. Abd-Ellah, and F. Yousef. 2011. "Female Genital Mutilation in Upper Egypt in the New Millennium." *International Journal of Gynaecology & Obstetrics* 114 (1): 47–50. doi:10.1016/j.ijgo.2011.02.003.

Silove, D., V. Manicavasagar, M. Coello, and J. Aroche. 2005. "PTSS, Depression, and Acculturation." *Intervention* 3: 46–50. http://www.ourmediaourselves.com/archives/31pdf/46_50 Silove.pdf.

Tinghog, P., and J. Carstensen. 2010. "Cross-Cultural Equivalence of HSCL-25 and WHO (ten) Wellbeing Index: Findings From a Population-Based Survey of Immigrants and Non-Immigrants in Sweden." *Community Mental Health Journal* 46: 65–76. doi:10.1007/s10597-009-9227-2.

UNICEF. 2004. Eradication of Female Genital Mutilation in Somalia. Advocacy paper. Geneva: The United Nations Children's Fund. Accessed September 27, 2011. http://www.unicef.org/somalia/SOM_FGM_Advocacy_Paper.pdf

UNICEF. 2005. *Female Genital Mutilation/Cutting. A Statistical Exploration*. Geneva: The United Nations Children's Fund. Accessed March 24, 2008. www.unicef.org/publications/index_29994.html

Vega, W., B. Kolody, and J. Valle. 2000. "Migration and Mental Health: An Empirical Test of Depression Risk Factors among Immigrant Mexican Women." *International Migration Review* 21: 512–530. doi:10.2307/2546608.

Vloeberghs, E., J. Knipscheer, A. Van der Kwaak, Z. Naleie, and M. Van den Muijsenbergh. 2011. *Veiled Pain. A Research in the Netherlands into the Psychological, Social and Relational Effects of Female Genital Mutilation*. Utrecht: Pharos. Accessed December 21, 2012. http://www.pharos.nl/documents/doc/webshop/veiled_pain.pdf.

WHO Study Group on Female Genital Mutilation and Obstetric Outcome. 2006. "Female Genital Mutilation and Obstetric Outcome: WHO Collaborative Prospective Study in Six African Countries." *Lancet* (367): 1835–1841. http://www.who.int/reproductivehealth/publications/fgm/fgm-obstetric-study-en.pdf.

WHO. 2012a. *Female Genital Mutilation*. Geneva: World Health Organization. Accessed December 14, 2012. http://www.who.int/topics/female_genital_mutilation/en/

WHO. 2012b. *Female Genital Mutilation. Factsheet No. 241*. Geneva: World Health Organization. Accessed December 14, 2012. http://www.who.int/mediacentre/factsheets/fs241/en/

Differences in working conditions and employment arrangements among migrant and non-migrant workers in Europe

Elena Ronda Pérez[a,b,c], Fernando G. Benavides[a,c,d], Katia Levecque[e], John G. Love[f], Emily Felt[a,d] and Ronan Van Rossem[e]

[a]CISAL, Research Centre in Occupational Health, Parc Recerca Biomèdica de Barcelona, Barcelona, Spain; [b]Public Health Area, Alicante University, Alicante, Spain; [c]CIBERESP, Madrid, Spain; [d]Pompeu Fabra University, Parc Recerca Biomèdica de Barcelona, Barcelona, Spain; [e]Ghent University, Ghent, Belgium; [f]Robert Gordon University, Aberdeen, UK

Objective. To determine migrant workers' exposure to select occupational risks and compare it with that of non-migrant workers in Europe.

Design. Based on the European Working Conditions Survey (EWCS-2005, $n = 29,654$ workers, 31 countries) we examined differential prevalence amongst migrant and non-migrant workers' primary paid jobs in terms of employment arrangements (working >10 hours/day, working >5 days/week, on Sundays, without a contract, changes in the work schedule and not free to decide when to take holidays or days off) and working conditions (exposure to hazards including chemical, physical agents, physical load and psychological conditions). For the purpose of this study, a migrant is defined as a person without nationality of the country of residence ($n = 926$). Adjusted prevalence ratios (aPRs) for age, economic sector and education were calculated.

Results. Differences in employment arrangements and working conditions were noted by migration status, gender and occupational status. Among non-manual workers, migrant males are more exposed than non-migrant males to negative psychosocial conditions – working at a very high speed (aPR 1.23; 95% CI 1.07–1.42) and shift work (aPR 1.66; 95% CI 1.27–2.17) – and adverse employment arrangements: working on Sundays (aPR 1.91; 95% CI 1.42–2.55), variable starting/finishing times (aPR 1.17; 95% CI 1.04–1.32) and changes in work schedule (aPR 1.56; 95% CI 1.30–1.88). Compared with non-migrant males, male migrant manual workers are the group with a greater number of disparities in terms of exposure to negative working conditions. Female migrant non-manual workers are more exposed to psychosocial conditions – working at very high speed (aPR 1.26; 95% CI 1.10–1.44) and shift work (aPR 1.61; 95% CI 1.29–2.01) while female manual migrant workers were more likely to report standing or walking (aPR 2.43; 95% CI 1.98–2.97), not having a contract (aPR 2.94; 95% CI 2.07–4.10) and not being free to decide days off and holidays (aPR 1.25; 95% CI 1.07–1.48) than non-migrants.

Conclusion. Migrant workers across Europe are more likely to be exposed to certain working and employment arrangements that may place them at higher risk of future health problems.

Introduction

People's relationship with work, their employment arrangements and the nature and conditions of that work influence health considerably. For most people, paid work is not only the main source of income, but also an important provider for other less tangible benefits related to health, such as self-esteem, social engagement and social prestige or recognition. Work can promote good physical and mental health, just as it can also have adverse effects on it because occupational settings are a source of exposure to environmental agents and conditions with potential negative effects on health (Nelson *et al.* 2005, Hämäläinen *et al.* 2009). Also, the ties that support the relationship between employer and employee – contracts, vacations and permissions among others – make workers more vulnerable in unstable or unprotected jobs with a respective impact on their well-being (Benavides *et al.* 2000, Artazcoz *et al.* 2005). Data concerning European statistics on accidents at work for 2009 show that 3.2% of workers reported an accident at work, which would correspond to almost seven million workers. Moreover, 8.6% of workers experienced a work-related health problem (nearly 20 million individuals) (Eurostat 2009).

Searching for work has been one of the largest drivers of migration in the last decade with many people moving from poor to developing countries seeking employment opportunities. So far Europe is a preferred target area for migrants (Gijón-Sánchez *et al.* 2010). Approximately, 11.1% of the European workforce is foreign-born (OECD 2011). Additionally, there are an unknown number of irregular or undocumented migrants, believed to account from 0.4 to 0.8% of the population in the 27 EU member states (Vogel 2009).

Most migrants (documented and undocumented) to Europe are recruited for the most unqualified and flexible jobs, with unskilled occupations in the service sector currently representing the main source of employment for such movers. At the same time, foreign-born workers are disproportionately under-represented in the sectors of education and administration, which typically comprise occupations with more secure employment contracts and better working conditions. By contrast, agriculture, manufacturing and construction are likely and important sources of employment for migrants in almost all European countries (Münz 2007). However, the migrant labour market is a segmented labour market with gender defining markedly different sector experiences for men and women. Thus migrant women are mainly concentrated in the tertiary sector, in low-skilled jobs such as domestic service (including cleaning and childcare), hotel cleaning, waitressing and the sex industry, although some migrant women respond to labour demand for skilled jobs and work as nurses and other health care workers. They are also found in retail sales and in labour-intensive manufacturing (Rubin *et al.* 2008).

It has been suggested that it is the disproportionate representation of migrants in unregulated jobs that accounts for the higher rates of occupational injuries observed among migrant workers compared with non-migrants in studies carried out in Spain and Italy (Colao *et al.* 2006, Lopez-Jacob *et al.* 2008, Rubiales-Gutierrez *et al.* 2010). Two Nordic studies that compared native workers with migrant workers, where both groups performed the same type of regulated jobs, did not find differences in the proportion of injuries (Döös *et al.* 1994, Salminen *et al.* 2009). Also, it has been suggested that the type of contract may influence the rates of occupational injuries for migrants (Patussi *et al.* 2008), although the information concerning the migrant working population in Europe is very scarce, and further work is needed to confirm such a suspicion (Ahonen *et al.* 2007, González and Irastorza 2007). Furthermore, research is needed that can explore the difference in the pattern of exposure to occupational risks by sex and occupation among migrant and non-migrant workers.

Notwithstanding the paucity of research in the area, migrant status is a key cross-cutting mechanism linking employment and working conditions to health inequalities (Benach *et al.* 2011). Given the substantial number of migrant workers in Europe, and the possible social and occupational consequences that this holds, it is important to have more concrete information on the experiences of the migrant population in terms of workplace conditions and employment arrangements. The goal of this study was to measure, stratifying by sex, the prevalence of the exposure of migrant workers to occupational and employment risks and to compare it with that of the non-migrant population.

Methods

Data source

Data were obtained from the fourth European Working Conditions Survey (EWCS), a five-year investigation (conducted annually) into the working arrangements and experiences of those economically active across EU member states and partner countries. The sample of the EWCS is representative of people in employment (employees and self-employed) during the fieldwork period (between 19 September and 30 November 2005) in each of the 31 countries included (all EU25 Member States plus Bulgaria, Croatia, Norway, Romania, Turkey and Switzerland). The EWCS is based upon a multi-stage, stratified and clustered sampling design, and this survey, with the exception of Belgium, Sweden, Netherlands and Switzerland (where telephone contact was used), employed a 'random walk' procedure for the selection of the respondents at the final stage. The latter procedure for the selection of respondents followed a strictly pre-defined approach. Starting from an assigned address within a designated area (defined geographically and by level of urbanisation), the interviewer was directed to choose every third building to the left of the address to identify a potential sampling unit. Once a household was selected, it could not be substituted even if there was nobody at home, until four attempts to contact the interviewee had been unsuccessful (at different times and days). The 'random walks' were scheduled at a time of the day when the employees and self-employed were available (normally, in the evenings and weekends) (Eurofound 2005). Using this method, 1000 interviews were sought in each of the participating countries (with the exception of Cyprus, Estonia, Luxembourg, Malta and Slovenia where 600 were sought). In total, 72,300 households were visited and 29,766 respondents were interviewed face-to-face (Jettinghoff and Houtman 2009, Niedhammer *et al.* 2012). Survey participation was measured in three separate ways: the cooperation rate (i.e., the proportion of interviews carried out to all eligible sampling units contacted), the contact rate (i.e., the proportion of all contacted households to all eligible households) and the response rate (i.e., the proportion of completed interviews to the total number of eligible respondents). The respective 'scores' on each measure were 66, 80 and 48% (Eurofound 2005), indicating generally high levels of cooperation by respondents although variable rates of participation were noted across countries. With respect to the latter, three countries (i.e., Belgium, Switzerland and Netherlands) which opted for telephone contact by way of screening respondents (rather than the 'random walk' procedure) reported the lowest 'response' rates overall at 34, 32 and 28%, respectively, whilst four countries (i.e., Czech Republic, Portugal, Romania and Spain) adopting the 'random walk' reported rates of 66% or higher (Eurofound 2005).

For the purposes of the study, employed persons were defined as people aged 15 years and older, having any paid job during the reference week or who had a job but were temporarily absent. Response rate ranged from Czech Republic (67%) to Netherlands (28%). Detailed information about the fieldwork is provided elsewhere (Eurofound 2005).

Occupational exposure information

The questionnaire gathered information about respondents' employment and working conditions related to the main paid job (the one where she/he spent more hours). For the purpose of this study we selected those with prevalence higher than 10%. The employment arrangements were evaluated by six questions: presence (yes/ no) of working without having a contract, working with fixed starting and finishing times, regular changes in the work schedule, working at least one Sunday per month, and working regularly more than 10 hours a day in a month.

Additionally, a series of items referred to working conditions, chemicals (breathing fumes, dust or powders), physical agents (noise, vibrations, extreme temperatures), physical load (tiring or painful positions, carrying or moving heavy loads, standing or walking, repetitive hand or arm movements) and psychosocial conditions (working at very high speed and shift work), were included. Frequency (seven-level rating scales from never to always) of these exposures was reported. A worker was considered to be exposed to each risk when he/she reported it as being present more than half of the time in a normal working day. Exposure to shift work was explored using a specific question that was translated into a binary variable (yes/no).

Migrant status and other variables

Migrant status was used as the main explanatory variable. According to the available information in the questionnaire, migrant is a person who is not a national of the country where the survey was being carried out. Workers with incomplete data in this variable ($n = 35$) were excluded.

Other selected variables were socio-demographic characteristics, i.e., sex, age (<24, 25–39, 40–54 and >55 years) and education (highest level completed by the respondent and grouped into the following categories: no education, primary, secondary and university), economic sector (defined as the main activity of the company or organisation: agriculture, manufacturing, construction and services) and occupation (manual and non-manual). The occupation reported in the EWCS was obtained from the question 'What is the title of your main paid job?' This information was classified according to the broad groups used in the International Standard Classification of Occupation (ISCO). This classification uses the criteria of skill to define the first level of occupational group: those occupations that require a similar level of skill form part of the same broad group; non-manual workers (administrators, managers, technicians and associate professionals, clerks, personal and protective service workers, sales occupations and skilled workers) and manual workers (semi-skilled and unskilled workers).

Data analysis

Men and women were analysed separately. Socio-demographic and labour characteristics were described by migrant status. Prevalence of self-reported exposure to working and employment arrangements in migrant and non-migrant workers was calculated. We performed chi-squared tests to examine the differences in proportions of all the variables in both groups. The measure of association between migrant status and exposure was the prevalence ratio (PR) with its 95% confidence interval (95% CI), calculated by generalised linear models crude and adjusted by age, educational level and economic sector. These analyses were performed separately by occupation. The software used was Statistical Package for the Social Sciences 19.0.

Results

Table 1 provides a socio-demographic profile of the sample. In terms of age, migrants were younger than non-migrants, with three-fifths of migrants aged 39 years or

Table 1. Description of the study population. European Working Conditions Survey, 2005.

| Characteristics | Male | | | | Female | | |
| | Non-migrants ($n=16,428$) | Migrants ($n=502$) | | | Non-migrants ($n=12,300$) | Migrants ($n=424$) | |
	n (%)	n (%)	p		n (%)	n (%)	p
Age (years)			<0.001				0.079
< 24	2087 (12.7)	65 (12.9)			1549 (12.6)	68 (16.0)	
25–39	5964 (36.3)	248 (49.4)			4696 (38.2)	170 (40.1)	
40–54	6174 (37.6)	161 (32.1)			4614 (37.5)	142 (33.5)	
> 55	2202 (13.4)	27 (5.6)			1440 (11.7)	44 (10.4)	
Educational level			0.018				<0.001
No education	212 (1.3)	10 (1.9)			166 (1.3)	17 (4.1)	
Primary education	1618 (9.8)	47 (9.4)			875 (7.1)	33 (7.9)	
Secondary education	10,940 (66.6)	310 (61.7)			7994 (64.9)	253 (59.6)	
University education	3658 (22.3)	135 (26.9)			3265 (26.7)	121 (28.4)	
Economic sector			<0.001				0.091
Services	8840 (53.8)	241 (48.0)			7975 (74.5)	258 (83.5)	
Manufacturing	1667 (10.2)	18 (3.6)			708 (5.8)	8 (1.9)	
Construction	4128 (25.1)	93 (18.5)			1800 (14.6)	38 (9.0)	
Agriculture	1793 (10.9)	150 (29.9)			220 (1.8)	5 (1.2)	
Occupation			<0.001				<0.001
No manual	9545 (58.1)	243 (48.4)			9665 (78.6)	271 (63.9)	
Manual	6883 (41.9)	259 (51.6)			2635 (21.4)	153 (36.1)	

younger compared with half or less of non-migrants similarly aged. With respect to education, more than four-fifths of both migrants and non-migrants had completed secondary or university studies, although differences by migration status and gender indicate that migrant women were more likely than other groups to have no education qualifications at all. Data on industrial sector highlight the segmented labour market experienced by migrant workers, one that is further differentiated by gender. Amongst men, migrants were concentrated in the primary and secondary sectors, especially in agriculture, whereas non-migrant men were more likely to be found in service sector employment, construction and manufacturing. Overall, women, both migrant and non-migrant, were more likely to be found in the tertiary sector, with migrant women especially likely to be in service sector employment. Within industrial sectors, migrant men were more evenly split between manual and non-manual occupations while the population of non-migrant men were more represented in non-manual occupations (58.1%). By contrast, nearly two-fifths of female migrants worked in manual occupations.

The prevalence of self-reported exposure to occupational health risks in migrants and non-migrants in Europe can be observed in Table 2. Male migrant workers show significantly higher prevalence in 8 of the 11 working conditions included, and in 4 of the 6 employment arrangements included. For female workers, the significant differences in working conditions relate to carrying or moving heavy things and standing or walking; both were higher amongst migrants. In relation to employment arrangements, there were differences in working on Sunday and not having a contract.

Taking non-migrant as a reference category, Table 3 shows the aPR associated with self-reported occupational exposures by occupational group (manual and non-manual) adjusting for age, educational level and economic sector. Non-manual migrant workers reported similar exposure to negative working conditions as did non-migrants, except for psychosocial agents – working at very high speed (aPR 1.23; 95% CI 1.07–1.42) and shift work (aPR 1.66; 95% CI 1.27–2.17). Most male migrant workers reported worse employment arrangements than non-migrants in terms of working on Sundays (aPR 1.91; 95% CI 1.42–2.55), variable starting/finishing times (aPR 1.17; 95% CI 1.04–1.32) and changes in the work schedule aPR 1.56 (95% CI 1.30–1.88). Most male migrant manual workers reported being exposed to more negative working conditions than their non-migrant counterparts, except for low temperatures, breathing fumes, dust or powders, and shift work, in which there are no differences. For all the negative employment arrangements surveyed there are no significant differences between migrants and non-migrants, except for variable starting/finishing times (aPR 1.08; 95% CI 1.00–1.17).

Exposure to negative working conditions for migrant female non-manual workers was more frequent than for non-migrants for noise (aPR 1.53; 95% CI 1.11–2.10), working at very high speed (aPR 1.26; 95% CI 1.10–1.44) and shift work (aPR 1.61; 95% CI 1.29–2.01) and more frequent for non-migrants: breathing fumes, dust or powders (aPR 0.17; 95% CI 0.06–0.52), trying or painful position (aPR 0.82; 95% CI 0.68–0.99) and carrying or moving heavy loads (aPR 0.67; 95% CI 0.46–0.97). Most non-manual migrant women reported more negative employment arrangements than non-migrants except for working on Sunday (aPR 1.30; 95% CI 1.09–1.56) and variable starting/finishing times (aPR 1.10; 95% CI 1.01–1.19). The significant

Table 2. Prevalence of self-reported exposure to occupational health risks in migrants and non-migrants in Europe. European Working Conditions Survey, 2005.

	Male			Female		
	Non-migrants (n = 16,428)	Migrants (n = 502)	p	Non-migrants (n = 12,300)	Migrants (n = 424)	p
Working conditions						
Vibrations from hand, tools, machinery	24.3	33.9	<0.001	7.2	10.1	0.026
Noise so loud that you have to raise your voice to talk to people	25.5	32.9	<0.001	12.3	13.9	0.373
High temperature which make you perspire	20.0	26.7	<0.001	11.4	13.0	0.362
Low temperatures, indoors or outdoors	17.1	16.3	0.693	7.7	9.4	0.212
Breathing fumes, dust or powders	20.4	22.1	0.378	6.9	3.8	0.017
Tiring or painful position	35.1	42.6	<0.001	30.6	34.0	0.151
Carrying or moving heavy loads	27.9	34.3	0.002	13.6	24.8	<0.001
Standing or walking	62.7	73.1	<0.001	58.4	69.8	<0.001
Repetitive hand or arm movement	51.5	63.1	<0.001	53.0	57.5	0.074
Working at very high speed	49.9	60.6	<0.001	46.0	45.8	0.976
Shift work	15.7	17.9	0.199	16.6	19.1	0.188
Employment arrangements						
Working on Sunday	33.1	29.1	0.067	25.4	31.6	<0.001
Working >10 hours/day	43.8	41.0	0.24	24.4	24.3	0.994
Variable starting/finishing times	55.0	63.1	<0.001	65.5	67.5	0.436
Not having a contract	7.4	10.0	0.04	7.5	17.0	<0.001
Changes in the work schedule	18.3	25.7	<0.001	18.0	21.0	0.128
Not free to decide days off or holidays	47.3	55.6	<0.001	50.6	54.5	0.130

differences of exposure in working conditions in manual migrant and non-migrant women workers were for standing or walking (aPR 2.43; 95% CI 1.98–2.97) – more reported by migrants – and exposure to noise (aPR 0.54; 95% CI 0.35–0.85); breathing fumes, dust or powders (aPR 0.37; 95% CI 0.18–0.77) and shift work aPR 0.53 (95% CI 0.34–0.85) were more reported by non-migrants. In terms of employment arrangements there were no significant differences in non-migrants

Table 3. Association of self-reported exposure with occupational health risks in migrants and non-migrants in Europe. European Working Conditions Survey, 2005.

| | Male | | Female | |
| | Non-manual | Manual | Non-manual | Manual |
	aPR (95% CI)[a]	aPR (95% CI)[a]	aPR (95% CI)[a]	aPR (95% CI)[a]
Working conditions				
Vibrations	1.04 (0.73–1.48)	1.37 (1.23–1.53)	1.02 (0.57–1.81)	0.89 (0.61–1.30)
Noise	0.71 (0.47–1.06)	1.40 (1.26–1.56)	1.53 (1.11–2.10)	0.54 (0.35–0.85)
High temperature	0.84 (0.58–1.21)	1.40 (1.21–1.63)	0.92 (0.63–1.35)	0.96 (0.67–1.38)
Low temperatures, indoors or outdoors	0.40 (0.22–0.73)	1.06 (0.85–1.32)	1.18 (0.80–1.75)	0.88 (0.50–1.52)
Breathing fumes, dust or powders	0.76 (0.48–1.19)	0.99 (0.83–1.18)	0.17 (0.06–0.52)	0.37 (0.18–0.77)
Tiring or painful position	0.83 (0.65–1.06)	1.35 (1.19–1.53)	0.82 (0.68–0.99)	1.00 (0.84–1.20)
Carrying or moving heavy loads	0.92 (0.64–1.30)	1.30 (1.16–1.47)	0.67 (0.46–0.97)	2.43 (1.98–2.97)
Standing or walking	1.18 (0.98–1.30)	1.12 (1.07–1.17)	0.89 (0.63–1.03)	1.02 (0.92–1.14)
Repetitive hand or arm movement	1.05 (0.91–1.22)	1.28 (1.21–1.36)	0.94 (0.84–1.06)	1.01 (0.92–1.11)
Working very high speed	1.23 (1.07–1.42)	1.23 (1.11–1.37)	1.26 (1.10–1.44)	1.01 (0.85–1.21)
Shift work	1.66 (1.27–2.17)	0.83 (0.62–1.10)	1.61 (1.29–2.01)	0.53 (0.34–0.85)
Employment arrangements				
Working on Sunday	1.91 (1.42–2.55)	0.83 (0.64–1.07)	1.30 (1.09–1.56)	1.29 (0.99–1.68)
Working >10 h/day	1.08 (0.96–1.22)	0.73 (0.59–0.91)	1.04 (0.84–1.29)	1.09 (0.77–1.53)
Variable starting/finishing times	1.17 (1.04–1.32)	1.08 (1.00–1.17)	1.10 (1.01–1.19)	0.93 (0.82–1.05)
Not having a contract	0.85 (0.50–1.45)	1.31 (0.91–1.89)	0.66 (0.42–1.03)	2.94 (2.07–4.10)
Changes in the work schedule	1.56 (1.30–1.88)	0.91 (0.73–1.14)	0.99 (0.78–1.27)	1.26 (0.95–1.69)
Not free to decide days off or holidays	1.16 (0.95–1.05)	1.14 (0.98–1.32)	1.00 (0.83–1.21)	1.25 (1.07–1.48)

aPR, adjusted prevalence ratio; 95% CI, 95% confidence interval.
[a]aPR for age, educational level and economic sector. In all categories non-migrants are the reference category (1.00).

and migrants, though not having a contract (aPR 2.94; 95% CI 2.07–4.10), and not free to decide days off or holidays (aPR 1.25; 95% CI 1.07–1.48) was more frequent in migrants.

Discussion

This is the first secondary analysis of the EWCS presenting the prevalence of exposure to different categories of working conditions and employment arrangements in migrant and non-migrant workers across Europe. Despite the heterogeneity of the finding, some patterns can be highlighted; migrant male and female non-manual workers are more exposed than non-migrants to adverse psychosocial conditions and to some adverse employment arrangements. Manual male migrant workers are the group with the greatest number of disparities in exposure to negative working conditions compared with those of non-migrants. For female migrant manual workers, the likelihood of working without a contract increases nearly threefold.

With regard to migrant workers' higher exposure to adverse working conditions, it has previously been documented that migrants face great difficulties in entering the labour market, and this can contribute to their occupying the most hazardous jobs (European Foundation for the Improvement of Living and Working Conditions 2007, González and Irastorza 2007, Münz 2007, Benach *et al.* 2011). Shortages in the local labour supply for certain unskilled occupations, and – on the part of migrant workers – poor language skills, poor knowledge of the labour market, less efficient job-seeking strategies compared to native workers and difficulties in validating prior educational and technical training (e.g., university degrees) in the host country might explain these results.

However, for women, no such differences were found between non-migrant and migrant women, and migrant women even report less exposure to negative working conditions. This absence of differences between migrant and non-migrant women workers could be in part related to female labour market segregation; the fact that women are more highly concentrated in fewer types of jobs than men, and that migrant and native women tend to be employed in similar kinds of jobs, especially those which are unskilled (Rubin *et al.* 2008). It could also be possible that, although we controlled for socio-demographic variables, the subjective value of the reported exposure could differ in migrant and non-migrant populations. In a qualitative study of occupational risks in migrant workers in Spain, women often seemed quite ambivalent in discussing their working conditions, especially with regard to potential hazards. When given examples of things they might have experienced at work, some women reported being exposed to the same physical load and chemicals in their jobs as in their unpaid work, where they were not perceived as hazards (Ahonen *et al.* 2009). Similarly, a Danish study showed that non-Western immigrant cleaners reported a better psychosocial work environment than Danish cleaners (Olesen *et al.* 2011). The authors suggested that migrants might have lower expectations of their working environment, and this may result in higher satisfaction. This might also be influenced by cultural differences and the perceived freedom (or lack thereof) to express comments critical of working conditions and the employer; eventhough the questionnaire was anonymous.

Over the last two decades, a large number of empirical studies have highlighted the impact of work-related psychosocial risk factors on physical and mental health outcomes (Bambra 2011). Workers exposed to these factors are at an increased risk of developing cardiovascular diseases (Rosengren et al. 2004), metabolic syndrome (Chandola et al. 2006), musculoskeletal symptoms (Bongers et al. 1993) and mental disorders (Stansfeld et al. 1999). Our study has shown that in non-manual migrant workers the frequency of exposure to negative working conditions was similar with the exception of the less favourable psychosocial environment for migrant workers. This result coincides with that observed in other national working conditions surveys carried out in countries with different migratory profiles and which have included other dimensions of the psychosocial work environment such as work organisation, job contents and demands at work (McKay et al. 2006, Blom and Blom 2009). A study comparing psychosocial working conditions among Swedish- and foreign-born employed persons suggests that maybe Swedes leave jobs with poor psychosocial work environments for better jobs, while migrants remain in the same type of job because they have difficulties in moving on to better jobs. Another possibility may be that Swedes find it easier to advance to better jobs within the same company than do migrants (Sundquist et al. 2003).

A simple explanation cannot be provided for our findings related to employment arrangements. Most of the countries included in this analysis belong to the European Union, and they are subject to a national interpretation of the Working Time Directive 2003/88/EC. While this provides relatively weak regulation of total hours, rest breaks and holidays, specific national legislation and collective regulation can impose further constraints on working-time practices at the workplace level.

There are some methodological shortcomings to consider when looking at our findings. A first limitation is the small number of migrants surveyed (Eurostat estimates that migrants comprise around 7% of the European workforce but the survey included only around 3% of migrant workers) (Eurostat 2010), precluding the possibility of carrying out analyses by world region of origin (such as distinguishing between migrants from Europe or from low human development index countries). We cannot exclude the possibility that working and employment conditions differ significantly between migrant groups according to region of origin, e.g., those migrants originating from within or outside of Europe, or from different regions within the EU.

Second, the data are based on self-reported exposures by workers and cannot be compared with other objective measurements. There remain issues around the validity of comparing self-reported measures of working conditions and employment arrangements between different countries with distinct cultures, attitudes and regulations (Orrenius and Zavodny 2009). Third, the migrant sample might not be representative of migrant workers in Europe in general and give rise to a selected bias. Specifically, the undocumented could be under-represented. There are indications in national labour reports that individuals working illegally may be exposed to worse working conditions and employment arrangements and may experience more serious situations of discrimination and exploitation, thus the measures of associations could be underestimated. Fourth, nationality has been used as an indicator of migrant status. Nationality indicates citizenship and in our study therefore picks up relevant processes that are connected to variation in legal rights on the labour market, social security and the use of health care services. The use of nationality to differentiate migrants from non-migrants does, however, entail some limitations. For instance, migrants may take the nationality of the host country which can induce possible bias due to poor classification, e.g., where nationality has been acquired through marriage. In addition, nationality does not reveal information on the length of migrants' residence in the host country. Research has shown that the life and work situation of people recently arrived to the country is quite different from those who have been born or lived there for a long time, and this could also influence their knowledge of occupational risks (Schenker 2010). Another relevant limitation is that nationality may or may not overlap with ethnic identity or minority status, a factor that might be connected to working conditions, employment arrangements and health status. Research has not been able to throw a clear picture on this interconnectedness yet, but exclusion and discrimination based on colour, race or ethnicity have been identified as major factors influencing both labour market position and health status (e.g., Mladovsky 2007; Levecque *et al.* 2007; Ingleby 2009; Rechel *et al.* 2011). This possible overlap between nationality and ethnic identity might differ significantly between the 31 countries in our sample, since there are huge differences in both the size and composition of the migrant populations (Ingleby 2009). The dominant foreign groups within each country in Europe reflect the sources from which labour has been recruited since WWII, historical linked and bilateral relations with former colonies, and ease of access (in terms of geography or policy) for refugees and asylum seekers from different places (Salt 2011). As the EWCS does not allow identification of ethnicity, or region of origin or other correlated features, it does not allow us to look into this matter in more depth. However, information on both nationality and belonging to an ethnic minority group is available for 41,677 respondents in 25 countries taking part in the European Social Survey 2006–2007. Analyses of this ESS data (results not shown) reveal that in the non-Eastern European countries and in general, about one or two non-nationals in five consider themselves to belong to an ethnic minority group. Of those reporting ethnic minority status, about two-thirds have (obtained) the nationality of the country of residence. In Eastern Europe, the pattern is quite different: quasi all respondents report themselves as nationals, even those of an ethnic minority group. Exception to this rule is Estonia, where a large ethnic minority group does not have the Estonian nationality. Although these ESS data only lift a very small corner of the veil, they do indicate that the overlap between nationality and ethnicity differs considerably across European countries. For our study on occupational health, this finding suggests that there might be a significant cross-national variation in the overlap or interaction between causal mechanisms linked to nationality and those linked to ethnicity.

Fifth, a limitation recognised in the EWCS is the difference in the response rate between countries, which could lead to biased estimations. In order to avoid before analysing the databases we applied the non-response weighting. This weight was available at the databases and was built taking into account some key variables so that the bias of non-response was minimised. Obviously, that required knowing the real population figures for the variables used for producing these non-response weights; in this case, it was assumed that the figures of the European Labour Force Survey (LFS) were the real figures, to generate a weight that adjusts these results to the results of the LFS for the following variables: sex, age, region, occupation and economic activity. The method followed to calculate these weights was the raking method, which carries out an iterative process of estimation of the weights that would be required for each case in order to replicate with the survey data the marginals of the LFS in terms of the weighting variables (Eurofound 2005).

Finally, the EWCS survey was conducted at the end of an economic cycle characterised by high rates of employment. Accordingly, it will be interesting to see if these findings have changed since the current economic crisis which has caused shrinkage of the labour market, particularly in the construction and services sectors employing most of immigrant workers in Europe (Eurostat 2010).

The overall falls in fertility and a decline in mortality have led to a re-configuration of populations across Europe and have resulted in a chronic reduction in the proportion of economically active people across the community. Such demographic trends, coupled with demands for labour within countries experiencing advanced modernity, mark a significant milestone in the 'migration cycle' (IDEA 2009) of both western and northern European states (e.g., Germany, France and UK) and southern European states (e.g., Italy, Spain, Greece and Portugal) and have significant implications for the economic, social and cultural life of people across the EU and its partner countries. Of particular note will be the reduction in the proportion of (resident) workers to finance social expenditures (e.g., the welfare states) and the shortage of labour in key sectors, including social care, food processing, cleaning, as well as jobs in hi-tech job industries and engineering (Adebahr 2010).

In this context, sustained and well-managed migration will be required to meet the needs of the European labour market and ensure the region's future prosperity. Management of migration in order to optimise outcomes for migrants and facilitate their integration and contribution to receiving economies is also about ensuring social cohesion, inclusion and equity across Europe. It would be desirable to conduct research targeting these groups in order to elucidate the factors that could affect health as well as occupational safety, injury and work-related diseases prevention, among others.

Future research should incorporate methodological approaches that make it possible to study social, cultural and geographical variables that have not been considered to date and which may influence the working and employment exposure in both migrants and non-migrants. The next EWCS will help to monitor this situation and confirm these findings. For that the EWCS should be reviewed in order to include a representative sample of migrant workers and several migration-related indicators that help us to unravel the different determinants and mechanisms leading up to occupational health inequalities. Within this context, the EWCS might benefit especially from simultaneously including indicators on nationality, ethnicity, country of birth (of oneself and parents) and length of residence. In order to capture new migration flows and forms connected to the labour market, the EWCS would also benefit from paying explicit attention to the now widespread circulation of people in informal and short-term movements (Salt 2011) as it might be questioned whether these migrants are at specific risks of occupational health. In any case, the EWCS should consider the drawbacks of not including sufficient migration-related indicators in the survey, and the fact that the included indicators have been changed over time and are not always translated accurately into the different participating countries. This does not only hinder valid cross-national comparisons, but also the pooling of EWCS surveys organised in different years. Such pooling results in larger migrant samples thereby enabling researchers to study the heterogeneity within the migrant population (Levecque *et al.*2012).

In summary, migrants are an increasingly valuable economic and cultural resource across Europe but are more likely to be exposed to adverse working conditions and employment arrangements that may place them at increased risk for health problems. In particular, special attention must be paid to the circumstances and plight of male migrant manual workers, while the experience of female migrant non-manual workers needs to be better understood and monitored.

Key messages

- Findings suggest that migrant workers across Europe, especially manual, are more likely to be exposed to certain negative working conditions and employment arrangements.
- Further research based on internationally standardised survey data is required to explore the underlying differences across Europe and should incorporate methodological approaches that make it possible to study social, cultural, geographical variables that have not been considered to date and which may explicate the potential risks associated with working conditions and employment arrangements amongst both migrant and non-migrant workers.

References

Adebahr, C., 2010. Young leader group on the future of Europe: demographic trends, migration and social cohesion. *In: Report, Third Conference, American Council on Germany* [online], 1–6 June 2010, Brussels & Paris. Available from: http://www.draeger-stiftung.de/fileadmin/user_upload/konferenzen_2010/Report_Brussels-Paris_2010.pdf [Accessed 11 April 2012].

Ahonen, E.Q., Benavides, F.G., and Benach, J., 2007. Immigrant populations, work and health – a systematic literature review. *Scandinavian Journal of Work Environment & Health*, 33 (2), 96–104.

Ahonen, E.Q., *et al.*, 2009. A qualitative study about immigrant workers' perceptions of their working conditions in Spain. *Journal of Epidemiology & Community Health*, 63 (11), 936–942.

Artazcoz, L., *et al.*, 2005. Social inequalities in the impact of flexible employment on different domains of psychosocial health. *Journal of Epidemiology & Community Health*, 59 (9), 761–767.

Bambra, C., 2011. *The psychosocial work environment and risks to health. Work, worklessness, and the political economy of health.* Oxford: Oxford University Press.

Benach, J., *et al.*, 2011. Migration and "low-skilled" workers in destination countries. *PLoS Medicine*, 8 (6), e1001043.

Benavides, F.G., *et al.*, 2000. How do types of employment relate to health indicators? Findings from the second European survey on working conditions. *Journal of Epidemiology & Community Health*, 54 (7), 494–501.

Bongers, P.M., *et al.*, 1993. Psychosocial factors at work and musculoskeletal disease. Scandinavian Journal of Work. *Environment & Health*, 19 (5), 297–312.

Blom, S. and Blom, K., 2009. *Living conditions among immigrants in Norway 2005/2006.* Available from: www.ssb.no/english/subjects/rapp_200902_en.pdf [Accessed 8 October 2011].

Chandola, T., Brunner, E., and Marmot, M., 2006. Chronic stress at work and the metabolic syndrome: prospective study. *British Medical Journal (Clinical Research Ed.)*, 332 (7540), 521–525.

Colao, A.M., *et al.*, 2006. Occupational accidents among immigrant workers in the fabriano areas. *Medicina delLavoro*, 97 (6), 787–798.

Döös, M., Laflamme, L., and Backström, T., 1994. Immigrants and occupational accidents: a comparative study of the frequency and types of accidents encountered by foreign and Swedish citizens at an engineering plant in Sweden. *Safety Science*, 18 (1), 15–32.

Eurofound, 2005. *European working conditions survey* [online]. Available from: http://www.eurofound.europa.eu/ewco/surveys/ewcs2005/index.htm [Accessed 8 August 2011].

European Foundation for the Improvement of Living and Working Conditions, 2007. *Employment and working conditions of migrant workers* [online]. Available from: http://www.eurofound.europa.eu/ewco/studies/tn0701038s/ [Accessed 8 September 2011].

Eurostat, 2009. *Results from the labour force survey 2007 ad hoc module on accidents at work and work-related health problems* [online]. Available from: http://epp.eurostat.ec.europa.eu/portal/page/portal/eurostat/home [Accessed 8 September 2011].

Eurostat, 2010. *Population data* [online]. Available from: http://epp.eurostat.ec.europa.eu/portal/page/portal/population/data/main_tables [Accessed 8 September 2011].

Gijón-Sánchez, M., *et al.*, 2010. Better health for all in Europe. *Eurohealth*, 16 (1), 17–20.

González, E.R. and Irastorza, X., 2007. *Literature study on migrant workers* [online]. Available from: http://osha.europa.eu/literature_reviews/migrant_workers [Accessed 8 September 2011].

Hämäläinen, P., Saarela, K.L., and Takala, J., 2009. Global trend according to estimated number of occupational accidents and fatal work-related diseases at region and country level. *Journal of Safety Research*, 40 (2), 125–139.

IDEA, 2009. *Working Paper Europe: the continent of immigrants – trends, structures and policy implications*. Available from: http://www.idea6fp.uw.edu.pl/pliki/WP13_Europe_continent_of_migrants.pdf [Accessed 11 April 2012].

Ingleby, D., 2009. European research on migration and health. Background paper developed within the framework of the IOM project. *Assisting Migrants and Communities (AMAC): analysis of social determinants of health and health inequalities*. Geneva: International Organization of Migration.

Jettinghoff, K. and Houtman, I., 2009. A sector perspective on working conditions. *European foundation for the improvement of living and working conditions*. Available from: http://www.eurofound.europa.eu/pubdocs/2008/14/en/1/ef0814en.pdf [Accessed 9 April 2012].

Levecque, K., Lodewyckx, I., and Vranken, J., 2007. Depression and generalized anxiety in the general population in Belgium: a comparison between native and migrant groups. *Journal of Affective Disorders*, 97 (1–3), 229–239.

Levecque, K., *et al.*, 2012.Use of existing health information systems for migrant health research in Europe: challenges and opportunities. *In*: D. Ingleby, A. Krasnik, V. Lorant, and O. Razum, eds. *COST series on health and diversity, Volume 1: health inequalities and risk factors among migrants and ethnic minorities*. Antwerp and Apeldoorn: Garant Publishers, 53–68.

Lopez-Jacob, M.J., *et al.*, 2008. Occupational injury in foreign workers by economic activity and autonomous community (Spain 2005). *Revista Española de Salud Publica*, 82 (2), 179–187.

McKay, S., Craw, M., and Chopra, D., 2006. *Migrant workers in England and Wales. An assessment of migrant worker health and safety risks*. Norwich: Health and Safety Executive.

Mladovsky, P., 2007. *Migration and health in the EU*. Research note. Brussels: European Commission – Directorate-General Employment, Social Affairs and Equal Opportunities. Unit E1-Social and Demographic Analysis.

Münz, R., 2007. *Migration, labor markets, and integration of migrants: an overview for Europe* [online]. Available from: http://siteresources.worldbank.org/SOCIALPROTECTION/Resources/SP-Discussion-papers/Labor-Market-DP/0807.pdf [Accessed 18 November 2011].

Niedhammer, I., *et al.*, 2012. Exposure to psychosocial work factors in 31 European Countries. *Occupational Medicine*, 62 (3), 196–202.

Nelson, D.I., *et al.*, 2005. The global burden of selected occupational diseases and injury risks: methodology and summary. *American Journal of Industrial Medicine*, 48 (6), 400–418.

OECD, 2011. *Foreign and foreign-born labour force in OECD countries* [online]. http://www.oecd.org/document/30/0,3746,en_2649_37415_48326878_1_1_1_37415,00.htm [Accessed 9 September 2011].

Olesen, K., *et al.*, 2011. Psychosocial work environment among immigrant and Danish cleaners. *International Archives of Occupational and Environmental Health*, 85 (1), 89–95.

Orrenius, P.M. and Zavodny, M., 2009. Do immigrants work in riskier jobs? *Demography*, 46 (3), 535–551.

Patussi, V., *et al.*, 2008. Comparison of the incidence rate of occupational injuries among permanent, temporary and immigrant workers in friuli-venezia giulia. *Epidemiologia E Prevenzione*, 32 (1), 35–38.

Rechel, B., *et al.*, 2011. Migration and health in the European Union: an introduction. *In*: B. Rechel, *et al.*, eds. *Migration and health in the European Union*. Berkshire: Open University Press, McGraw-Hill, 3–13.

Rosengren, A., *et al.*, 2004. Association of psychosocial risk factors with risk of acute myocardial infarction in 11119 cases and 13648 controls from 52 countries (the INTERHEART study): case-control study. *Lancet*, 364 (9438), 953–962.

Rubiales-Gutierrez, E., *et al.*, 2010. Differences in occupational accidents in Spain according to the worker's country of origin. *Salud Publica de Mexico*, 52 (3), 199–206.

Rubin, J., *et al.*, 2008. *Migrant women in the EU labour force* [online]. Available from: http://ec.europa.eu/social/BlobServlet?docId=2098&langId=en [Accessed 28 September 2012].

Salminen, S., Vartia, M., and Giorgiani, T., 2009. Occupational injuries of immigrant and Finnish bus drivers. *Journal of Safety Research*, 40 (3), 203–205.

Salt, J., 2011. Trends in Europe's international migration. *In*: B. Rechel, *et al.*, eds. *Migration and health in the European Union*. Berkshire: Open University Press, McGraw-Hill, 17–36.

Schenker, M.B., 2010. A global perspective of migration and occupational health. *American Journal of Industrial Medicine*, 53 (4), 329–337.

Stansfeld, S.A., *et al.*, 1999. Work characteristics predict psychiatric disorder: prospective results from the Whitehall II Study. *Occupational and Environmental Medicine*, 56 (5), 302–307.

Sundquist, J., *et al.*, 2003. Psychosocial working conditions and self-reported long-term illness: a population-based study of Swedish-born and foreign-born employed persons. *Ethnicity & Health*, 8 (4), 307–317.

Vogel, D., 2009. Size and development of irregular migration to the EU. *Clandestino research project* [online]. Available from: http://irregular-migration.hwwi.de/typo3EN/Comparative PolicyBrief_SizeOfIrregularMigration_Clandestino_Nov09_2.pdf [Accessed 20 September 2011].

Review of community-based interventions for prevention of cardiovascular diseases in low- and middle-income countries

Steven van de Vijver[a,b], Samuel Oti[a,b], Juliet Addo[c], Ama de-Graft Aikins[d,e] and Charles Agyemang[f]

[a]Department of Global Health, Academic Medical Centre, University of Amsterdam, Amsterdam Institute for Global Health and Development, Amsterdam, The Netherlands; [b]African Population and Health Research Center, Nairobi, Kenya; [c]London School of Hygiene and Tropical Medicine, Faculty of Epidemiology and Population Health, London, UK; [d]Regional Institute for Population Studies, University of Ghana, Legon, Ghana; [e]LSE Health, London School of Economics and Political Science, London, UK; [f]Department of Public Health, Academic Medical Centre, University of Amsterdam, Amsterdam, The Netherlands

Background. An increasing burden of cardiovascular disease (CVD) is occurring in low- and middle-income countries (LMICs) as a result of urbanisation and globalisation. Low rates of awareness and treatment of risk factors worsen the prognosis in these settings. Prevention of CVD is proven to be cost effective and should be the main intervention. Insight into prevention programmes in LMIC is important in addressing the rising levels of these diseases.
Objective. To evaluate the effectiveness of the community-based interventions for CVD prevention programmes in LMIC.
Design. A literature review with searches in the databases of PubMed, EMBASE, CINAHL, LILACS, African Index Medicus and Google Scholar between 1990 and May 2012.
Results. Twenty-six studies involving population-based and high-risk interventions have been included in this review. The content of the population intervention was mainly health promotion through media and health education, and the high-risk approach focused often on education of patients, training of health care providers and implementing treatment guidelines. A few studies had a single intervention on exercising or salt reduction. Most studies showed a significant reduction of cardiovascular risk ranging from lifestyle changes on diet, smoking and alcohol to biomedical outcomes like blood pressure, glucose levels or weight. Some studies showed improved management of risk factors like increased control of hypertension or adherence to medication.
Conclusion. There have been effective community-based programmes aimed at reducing cardiovascular risk factors in LMIC but these have generally been limited to the urban poor. Health education with a focus on diet and salt, training of health care providers and implementing treatment guidelines form key elements in successful programmes.

Background

Cardiovascular diseases (CVDs) are the leading cause of mortality worldwide (Lopez et al. 2006). More than 80% of the global CVD deaths occur in low- and middle-income countries (LMICs), and this percentage is projected to increase even further in the next decade (WHO 2002, 2005, 2011). It is therefore anticipated that in the coming years, the burden of CVD could aggravate the already stretched and poorly responsive health systems of LMICs.

The increasing burden of CVDs is mainly driven by globalisation, westernisation, industrialisation and urbanisation (Godfrey and Julien 2005). These trends are strongly linked with changes in individual and societal lifestyle such as tobacco use, alcohol consumption, reduced physical activity and adoption of 'Western' diets that are high in salt, refined sugar and unhealthy fat and oils. These lifestyle factors have been demonstrated to be strong behavioural risk factors for CVD (Godfrey and Julien 2005). Overall, LMICs are experiencing rising trends in both behavioural and physiological risk factors for CVD with increasing urbanisation. Several studies have demonstrated that in urban settings, behavioural and physiological risk factors for CVD are higher than in rural areas (Addo, Smeeth, and Leon 2007; Agyemang 2006; Fuentes et al. 2000). Moreover, low rates of treatment and control of risk factors such as hypertension have been reported in LMICs, resulting in disproportionately higher morbidity and mortality rates (Addo, Smeeth, and Leon 2007; Walker et al. 2000).

Prevention of CVD risk has been shown to be both cost effective and scalable even in LMICs (WHO 2007). Additionally, focusing on the prevention and management of CVD risk factors will create more effective treatment, lower costs of care and reduce overall morbidity and mortality from CVD (Fuster and Kelly 2010). The Institute of Medicine Report on cardiovascular health in LMICs stresses the need for evidence and best practices for cost effective and sustainable community-based strategies for prevention and control of cardiovascular risk factors (Fuster and Kelly 2010).

Insight into prevention and control programmes for CVD is important in addressing the rising burden of these diseases. Previous interventions in high-income countries have been shown to have had positive outcomes, and lessons from these may be applicable to LMICs (Bhalla et al. 2006; Puska, Salonen, and Nissinen 1983). It is, however, important to know how these programmes can be implemented effectively in LMICs. It has been suggested that a structured, integrated programme is most effective in CVD prevention (Fuster and Kelly 2010). However, it is difficult to implement this in LMICs where capacity is low, health systems are poorly responsive and political will to effect necessary changes in policy might be lacking. Again, as funding and attention to prevention programmes of CVD in these regions has been limited over the years, it will be important for health planners and decision-makers to draw on best practices from other settings in the design of CVD prevention and control strategies in LMICs. Previously published studies on CVD control in LMICs (Gaziano, Galea, and Reddy 2007; WHO 2002, 2005, 2011) have often lacked practical real life application. It is essential to identify and evaluate effective strategies implemented in CVD prevention and control programmes in LMICs. Even if studies have focused on only a single risk factor they still might provide tools for new prevention programmes in these settings that are heavily needed.

Until now the intervention studies that have taken place in LMICs have not yet been evaluated. The main aim of this paper was, therefore, to assess the effectiveness of the population-based intervention studies for CVD prevention in LMIC. Our key research questions were (1) what kinds of community-based interventions on CVD prevention have been conducted in LMICs? (2) and which interventions were effective in reducing cardiovascular risk in LMIC?

Methods

We searched through the databases of PubMed, CINAHL, EMBASE, LILACS, African Index Medicus and Google Scholar for studies that were published between 1990 and the 1st of May 2012, and evaluated interventions of community-based prevention for CVD in LMICs among adults (≥ 18 years) with or without existing risk factors for CVD. The intervention had to be 'community-based'; meaning that the intervention was coordinated through worksites, schools, religious organisations, primary health care centres or other settings closely related to the participants in line with the American Heart Association Framework for public health practice for CVD prevention (Figure 1). Based on the American Heart Association Guide for Improving Cardiovascular Health at the Community Level (Pearson et al. 2003), we defined prevention of CVD as healthy lifestyle adjustments in order to reduce one or more risk behaviours (such as overweight or smoking) or screening and management of risk factors like hypertension and diabetes. We evaluated studies that compared intervention group with the control group without intervention, or compared the group before and after the intervention on any of the following outcomes: systolic and/or diastolic blood pressure, hypertension, glucose levels, HbA1c levels, body weight, body mass index (BMI), waist circumference, physical activity, salt intake, fat intake, smoking, alcohol intake and the rates of awareness, treatment and control of hypertension and diabetes. In addition, we evaluated other outcomes such as cost-effectiveness, feasibility and training on CVD prevention if this information was available. Because our focus was on community-based interventions, all studies on hospital-based intervention studies were excluded from this review.

In order to minimise bias from studies with small numbers of participants or short period of time we included only studies with ≥ 250 participants and follow-up period of minimum one year. Furthermore, non-English language published studies were excluded as there were no resources for accurate translations.

For this review, we defined 'medium to high risk group' as people having elevated blood pressure levels (blood pressure $\geq 140/90$ mmHg), elevated glucose levels (fasting glucose > 5.6 mmol/l or random blood sugars > 11.0 mmol/l) or overweight (BMI ≥ 25 Kg/m^2 or waist circumference > 102 cm among men and > 88 cm among women).

Results

Study characteristics

Twenty-six studies were included in this review (Figure 2). The overview of the articles is in Table 1. The selected studies were conducted between 1979 and 2008,

Essential Public Health Services

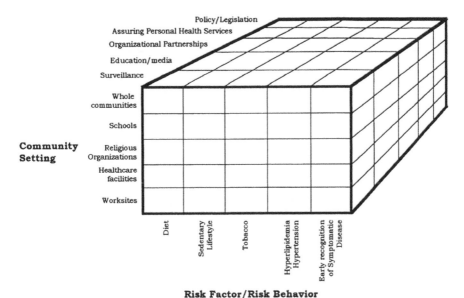

Figure 1. American Heart Association Framework for public health practice for CVD prevention. Reproduced with permission from Pearson et al. (2003).

and published between 1993 and 2011. The median sample size was 11,660 with a range from 284 (Gill et al. 2008) to 120,000 (Chen, Wu, and Gu 2008) participants and the length of follow-up varied between one year (Onat et al. 2003) and eight years (Chen, Wu, and Gu 2008). Most of the studies were conducted in urban or mixed urban and rural setting.

Twelve studies were based on population level, 3 studies focused on population level and medium or high risk groups and 11 studies focused on medium or high risk groups.

Among the 15 population-based studies there were national or regional programmes that included health promotion through media and approached the overall population with community programmes targeting schools, worksites and other public meeting places. Generally, these programmes aimed to raise knowledge, awareness and healthy behaviour at different levels such as diet, exercise, smoking and alcohol. Five population-based interventions focused on a specific risk factor like salt reduction (Cappuccio et al. 2006), diet adjustments (Almeida-Pittito et al. 2010) and exercising (Damião et al. 2010; Lara et al. 2008; Mohan et al. 2006). Three of the interventions (Chen, Wu, and Gu 2008; Lara et al. 2008) were strictly related to the worksite.

Among the 14 studies focusing on medium or high risk patients, most interventions involved providing health education to patients, training of health care staff and introduction of standardised treatment including guidelines. Two programmes studied outcomes of task shifting, mostly from doctor to nurses or clinical officers (Kengne et al. 2009; Gill et al. 2008) and one study (China Salt Substitute Study Collaborative Group 2007) concentrated only on implementation of salt substitution among medium or high risk patients.

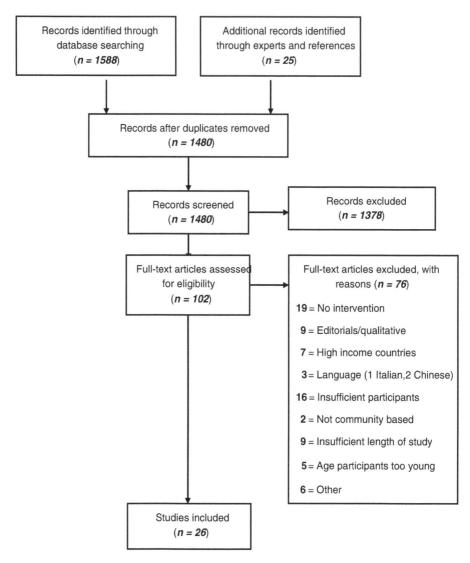

Figure 2. Study selection with flow based on the PRISMA 2009 Guidelines (Moher et al. 2009).

Study outcomes

In Table 2, there is an overview of the outcomes of the different studies with the same ranking of population-based intervention, mixed population and medium- or high-risk patients and finally only medium or high risk patients. Interventions were evaluated through different study designs including randomised control trial (Cappuccio et al. 2006; CSSS et al. 2007; Jafar et al. 2009; Ramachandran et al. 2006), cluster controlled trial (Harati et al. 2010), intervention trial (Chen, Wu, and Gu 2008; Huang et al. 2011; Kar et al. 2008; Khosravi et al. 2010; Sarrafzadegan et al. 2009), non-controlled experimental (Almeida-Pittito et al. 2010; Damião et al. 2010; Gill et al. 2008; Isaakidis et al. 2011; Kengne et al. 2009; Krishnan et al. 2011;

Table 1. Characteristics of included studies evaluating community-based interventions for prevention of CVD in LMIC.

Source	Location	Setting	Target	Period	Numbers	Age	Study design	Aim	Intervention
Almeida-Pittito et al. (2010)	Brazil	Urban	Population	2005–2007	394	60 years mean	Non-controlled experimental	Impact of lifestyle coaching on CVD risk factors	Health education and exercise trainings
Cappucio et al. (2006)	Ghana	Urban/ rural	Population	2001–2002	1013	55 years mean	Randomised control trial	Impact of education salt reduction on diet and BP	Health education + salt reduction
Chen, Wu, and Gu (2008)	China, Fangshan	Rural	Population	1991–1999	120,000	No data	Intervention trial	Impact of worksite intervention on CVD risk factors	Worksite screening, health education and management and surveillance
Chen, Wu, and Gu (2008)	China, Beijing	Urban	Population	1987–1995	110,000	No data	Intervention trial	Impact of worksite intervention on CVD risk factors	Worksite screening, health education and management and surveillance
Damião et al. (2010)	Brazil	Urban	Population	2005–2007	575	30 years <	Non-controlled experimental	Impact of nutritional advices on diets	Nutrition training on individual and group level
Dowse et al. (1995)	Mauritius	Urban/ rural	Population	1987–1992	5162	25–74 years	Cross-sectional surveys	Impact of lifestyle advices on CVD risk factors	Health promotion through media, health education worksite and schools

Table 1 (*Continued*)

Source	Location	Setting	Target	Period	Numbers	Age	Study design	Aim	Intervention
Krishnan et al. (2011)	India, Ballabgarh	Urban/ rural	Population	2004–2007	5143	41.5 years mean	Non-controlled experimental	Evaluation of health programme on CVD risk factors	Health promotion through media, health education, set-up clinic
Krishnan et al. (2011)	Indonesia	Urban	Population	2004–2007	1806	44.3 years mean	Non-controlled experimental	Evaluation of health programme on CVD risk factors	Health promotion through media, health education, set-up clinic
Lara et al. (2008)	Mexico	Urban	Population	2003–2004	335	18–87 years	Non-controlled experimental	Evaluate exercise training at work on CVD risk factors	Worksite exercise breaks
Mohan et al. (2006)	India, Chennai	Urban	Population	1998–2004	479	20 years <	Non-controlled experimental	Evaluate exercise programme on physical activity	Health promotion through media, health education
Sarrafzadegan et al. (2009)	Iran, Isfahan	Urban/ rural	Population	2000–2004	12515	18 years <	Intervention trial	Evaluation of health programme on CVD risk factors	Health promotion through media, health education, training health care

Table 1 (*Continued*)

Source	Location	Setting	Target	Period	Numbers	Age	Study design	Aim	Intervention
Yu et al. (1999)	China, Tianjin	Urban	Population	1989–1996	2000	15–64 years	Cross-sectional surveys	Evaluation of health programme on CVD risk factors	Health promotion through media + salt reduction
Huang et al. (2011)	China, Hubei	Urban/ rural	Population/ risk	2003–2006	1632	35 years <	Intervention trial	Evaluate effect of education on knowledge and CVD risk factors	Health education, training health care staff
Khosravi et al. (2010)	Iran, Isfahan	Urban/ rural	Population/ risk	2001–2007	12,514	18 years <	Intervention trial	Evaluate effect of treatment programme	Health promotion through media, health education, training health care
Rossouw et al. (1993)	South Africa	Rural	Population/ risk	1979–1983	7188	15–64 years	Cross-sectional surveys	Evaluation of health programme on CVD risk factors	Health promotion through media and health education
CSSS group (2007)	China, northern	Rural	Risk group	2004–2005	608	55 years <	Randomised control trial	Impact of salt substitutes on BP control	Introducing salt substitutes

Table 1 (*Continued*)

Source	Location	Setting	Target	Period	Numbers	Age	Study design	Aim	Intervention
Gill et al. (2008)	South Africa	Rural	Risk group	18 months	284	56 years mean	Non-controlled experimental	Evaluate nurse-led diabetes programme	Guidelines, training and patient education
Harati et al. (2010)	Iran, Teheran	Urban	Risk group	2002–2005	8212	20 years <	Cluster controlled trial	Impact of lifestyle modification on CVD risk factors	Intense health education (smoking, nutrition, exercise) among diabetes patients
Isaakidis et al. (2011)	Cambodia	Rural	Risk group	2002–2008	2858	18 years <	Non-controlled experimental	Describe and evaluate HT treatment programme	Health education and treatment
Jafar et al. (2009)	Pakistan	Urban	Risk group	2004–2007	4023	40 years <	Randomised control trial	Assess effect of treatment programme on BP and related risk factors	Health education households and training health care providers
Kar et al. (2008)	India, Haryana	Urban/rural	Risk group	2004–2005	1010	30 years <	Intervention trial	Assess feasibility of treatment programme	Training health care and guidelines
Kengne et al. (2009)	Cameroon	Urban/rural	Risk group	1998–2000	454	56 years mean	Non-controlled experimental	Describe and evaluate HT treatment programme	Guidelines and training nurses

Table 1 (*Continued*)

Source	Location	Setting	Target	Period	Numbers	Age	Study design	Aim	Intervention
Nguyen et al. (2011)	Vietnam	Rural	Risk group	2007–2008	497	25 years <	Non-controlled experimental	Describe and evaluate HT treatment programme	Hypertension Management Programme Health education, guidelines, training staff
Onat et al. (2003)	Turkey	Urban/ rural	Risk group	12 months	2012	40–70 years	Non-controlled experimental	Describe and evaluate HT treatment programme	Introducing guidelines for high risk patients
Ramachandran et al. (2006)	India	Urban/ rural	Risk group	2001–2004	531	35–55 years	Randomised control trial	Impact of lifestyle modification on prevention of diabetes	Mobile clinic, treatment and lifestyle advice
Salazar et al. (2005)	Argentina	Rural	Risk group	1997–2003	1377	15–75 years	Non-controlled experimental	Assess effect of treatment programme on BP and related risk factors	Health education, free medication

Table 2. Overview of results from selected studies.

Source	Blood pressure	Glucose/HbA1c	Weight reduction	Physical activity	Diet	Smoking	Manage risk factor
Almeida-Pittito et al. (2010)	No data available	Not significant	Reduction weight among 42%* participants pre vs post	Increase in physical activity among 7.4%* pre vs post	Reduction saturated fats in diet among 74.5%,* increase in fruit intake 39%* pre vs post	No data available	LTFU 2%
Cappuccio et al. (2006)	Reduction SBP 2.5 mmHg (-1.45 to 6.54), DBP 3.9 mmHg (0.78–7.11)* vs control[a]	No data available	No data available	No data available	No significant reduction in salt intake vs control	No data available	No data available
Chen, Wu, and Gu (2008) (rural)	Reduction in SBP 1.4 mmHg in men, 3.4 mmHg* in women vs control. DBP not significant	No data available	No data available	No data available	Reduction alcohol intake among men 10.4%* vs control	Reduction smoking among men 7.4%* vs control	No data available
Chen, Wu, and Gu (2008) (urban)	Reduction SBP 1.9 mmHg, reduction DBP 2.2 mmHg* vs control	No data available	No data available	No data available	Reduction in salt intake of 3.9 g/day* vs control	No data available	Increase in treatment of HT 46.3%,* increase control HT 34.5%* vs control

Table 2 (*Continued*)

Source	Blood pressure	Glucose/HbA1c	Weight reduction	Physical activity	Diet	Smoking	Manage risk factor
Damião et al. (2010)	Reduction among men in SBP 7.3 mmHg,** DBP 4.5 mmHg.** Reduction among women SBP 6.0 mmHg,** DBP 3.9mmHg** pre vs post	Reduction among men fasting glucose 7.21 mg/dl (4.72–9.71),** among women 3.73 mg/dl (1.71–5.75)*	Reduction among men in weight 0.9 kg (0.58–1.27)** and WC 2.03 cm (1.05–3.01), among women weight 0.4 kg (0.09–0.71),* WC 3.15 cm (2.54–3.76)* pre vs post	No significant increase in physical activity pre vs post	Reduction of fat intake among men 0.24 g/day (−3.96 to 4.45), among women 8.48 g/day (6.20–10.78),* alcohol reduction not significant pre vs post	No data available	No data available
Dowse et al. (1995)	Reduction among men in hypertension 2.9% (1.1–4.9),** among women 1.5% (0.0–3.0)*	No significant decrease pre vs post	Increase among men of obesity 1.9% (0.7–3.1),* among women 4.8% (3.0–6.6)*	Increase among men in activity 5.2% (2.9–7.5),** among women 1.4% (0.6–2.2)**	Reduction among men heavy alcohol consumption 23.8% (21.7–25.9),** among women 2.0% (1.3–2.7)**,b	Reduction among men 11.0% (8.1–13.9),** among women 3.2% (2.0–4.4)**,b	No data available
Krishnan et al. (2011; India)	Reduction among men in prevalence HT 8.6%,* SBP 2.1 mmHg,* DBP 1.2 mmHg,* among women prevalence HT 1.7%, SBP 2.6 mmHg,* DBP 1.0 mmHg pre vs post	No data available	Increase among men in prevalence overweight 0.2%, among women 2.0%	Reduction among men inactivity 3.0%, among women increase inactivity 18.3%*	Reduction among men in alcohol 1.7%, among women 0.1%. Increase among men in healthy diet 3.4%,* women 4.9%*	Reduction among men in smoking 0.8%, among women 1.6%	Increase among men in measurement of SBP in last year 6.4%,* and FBG 2.3%,* among women SBP 8.6%,* FBG 7.2%*

Table 2 (*Continued*)

Source	Blood pressure	Glucose/HbA1c	Weight reduction	Physical activity	Diet	Smoking	Manage risk factor
Krishnan et al. (2011; Indonesia)	Reduction among men in prevalence HT 5.2%,* SBP 13.8 mmHg,* DBP 7.5 mmHg,* among women prevalence HT 5.6%,* SBP 16.0 mmHg,* DBP 9.5 mmHg* pre vs post	No data available	Reduction among men overweight 11.5%,* reduction among women in WC 13.6%*	Reduction among men inactivity 3.9%, among women 19.2%*	Reduction among men in alcohol 3.3%, among women 0.3%. Increase among men in healthy diet 5.2%, among women 1.1%	Reduction among men in smoking 6.5%, among women 0%	Increase among men in measurement of SBP in last year 11.6%, and FBG 56.3%,* among women SBP 2.8%, FBG 62.1%*
Lara et al. (2008)	Increase among men SBP 0.1 mmHg, DBP 0.7 mmHg. Reduction among women SBP 1.0 mmHg, DBP 0.5 mmHg pre vs post	No data available	Reduction among men BMI 0.43* and waist circumference 1.9 cm,** among women BMI 0.25, waist circumference 1.4 cm*	No data available	No data available	No data available	No data available
Mohan et al. (2006)	No data available	No data available	No data available	Increase exercise 44.5% pre vs post*	No data available	No data available	No data available
Sarrafzadegan et al. (2009)	No data available	No data available	No data available	Decrease physical activity 0.6–9.6%*	Increase in healthy diet 17–21%,* in healthy lifestyle 30.5%*	Reduction in smoking 1.5–3.0% pre vs post	No data available

Table 2 (Continued)

Source	Blood pressure	Glucose/ HbA1c	Weight reduction	Physical activity	Diet	Smoking	Manage risk factor
Yu et al. (1999)	Reduction among men in prevalence in HT 2%,* SBP 0%, among women prevalence of HT 2%,* SBP 2 mmHg	No data available	Reduction among men in prevalence overweight 2%, among women 3%		Reduction in salt intake 6.0%	No data available	No data available
Huang et al. (2011)	Reduction prevalence HT 12.9%* pre vs post	No data available	No data available	Increase in exercise 16.4%* pre vs post	Reduction in alcohol 4.2%,* salt intake 30%,* fat intake 9.1%* pre vs post	Reduction in smoking 3.5% pre vs post	Increased knowledge on healthy lifestyle 6.6–55.5%,* increase awareness HT 18.5%,* treatment HT 12.7%,* control HT 24.3%* pre vs post
Khosravi et al. (2010)	Reduction in prevalence HT 3.3%** vs control. Reduction SBP 3.2 mmHg** pre and post	Reduction prevalence DM 0.8% vs control	Reduction BMI 2.5% vs control	No data available	No data available	No data available	Increase in awareness HT 9.4%,** treatment HT 8.9%,** control HT 8.7%**

Table 2 (*Continued*)

Source	Blood pressure	Glucose/HbA1c	Weight reduction	Physical activity	Diet	Smoking	Manage risk factor
Rossouw et al. (1993)	Reduction among men in SBP 4.5 mmHg (3.8–5.2),* DBP 2.3 mmHg (1.9–2.7),* among women SBP 6.3 mmHg (5.7–6.9),* DBP 3.4 mmHg (3.0–3.8)* pre vs post	No data available	Reduction among men in BMI 0.1 kg/m^2 (0.0–0.2), among women 0.5 kg/m^2 (0.4–0.6)*	No data available	No data available	Reduction among men in smoking 9.0% (7.2–10.8),* among women 5.2% (4.0–6.4)*	Increase among men in knowledge 7.5% (7.0–8.0),* among women 7.2% (6.8–7.7)*
CSSS group (2007)	Reduction SBP 5.4 mmHg (2.3–8.5),** DBP 0.7 mmHg (−0.5 to 1.9), pre vs post	No data available	No data available	No data available	No data available	No data available	No significant difference in treatment vs control, LTFU 2%
Gill et al. (2008)	No data available	Reduction in HbA1c 3.9%** pre vs post	Increase among men in BMI 2.2 kg/m^2,** among women 1.3 kg/m^2* pre vs post	No data available	No data available	No data available	LTFU 31%
Harati et al. (2010)	Reduction among men in SBP 3.2 mmHg (2.1–4.4)* and DBP 1.8 mmHg (0.6–3.0),* among women SBP 1.1 mmHg (0.1–2.0),* DBP 0.6 mmHg (0.03–1.2)*,c	Reduction among men in FBG 2.1 ml/dl (0.4–3.9),* among women 2.3 mg/dl (1.0–3.7)**	Reduction among men in weight 0.5 kg (0.1–0.9),* WC 0.2 cm (−0.6 to 1.0), among women weight 0.09 (−0.2 to 0.4), WC 1 cm (0.5–1.6)**,c	No data available	No data available	No data available	No data available

Table 2 (*Continued*)

Source	Blood pressure	Glucose/ HbA1c	Weight reduction	Physical activity	Diet	Smoking	Manage risk factor
Isaakidis et al. (2011)	Reduction in SBP 26 mmHg,** DBP 14 mmHg** pre vs post	No data available	No data available	No data available	No data available	No data available	Increase in control HT 36.5%* pre vs post, LTFU 42%
Jafar et al. (2009)	Reduction in SBP 10.8 mmHg (8.9–12.8),** DBP 4.7 mmHg* pre vs post[d]	No data available	No significant reduction in BMI	Increase in physical activity vs control group*	No data available	Reduction in smoking 2.8%** vs control	Increase in control of HT 29.6%** vs control, LTFU 22%
Kar et al. (2008)	Reduction in SBP 8.8 mmHg** pre vs post	No data available	Reduction in weight 0.55 kg	No data available	No data available	Increase of intention to quit smoking 49.0%** pre vs post	74.5% of referrals visit clinic, increase in control of HT 8.7%, increase in adherence 25.8%* pre vs post
Kengne et al. (2009)	Reduction in SBP 11.7 mmHg (8.9–14.4),** DBP 7.8 mmHg (5.9–9.7)** pre vs post	Reduction in FBG 1.4 mmol/L (0.6–2.6)* pre vs post	Reduction in weight 0.4 kg (0.1–0.8)* pre vs post	No data available	No data available	No data available	LTFU 88%
Nguyen et al. (2011)	Reduction in SBP 29.2–55.5 mmHg,* DBP 15.9–28.7 mmHg*	No data available	No data available	No data available	No data available	No data available	LTFU 34%
Onat et al. (2003)	Reduction SBP 26.0 mmHg (0.1–51.9 mmHg)*	No data available	No data available	No data available	No data available	Reduction smoking 18.2%* pre vs post	LTFU 53%

Table 2 (*Continued*)

Source	Blood pressure	Glucose/ HbA1c	Weight reduction	Physical activity	Diet	Smoking	Manage risk factor
Ramachandran et al. (2006)	No data available	15.5%* absolute risk reduction incidence DM vs control	No significant reduction in weight and WC	Increase physical activity 17.1%* pre vs post	Increase in healthy diet 19.1%* pre vs post	No data available	Increase in drug adherence 4.2% vs control, LTFU 4.9%
Salazar et al. (2005)	Reduction in SBP 5.5 mmHg,* DBP 6.9 mmHg* pre vs post	No data available	Reduction in weight 0.2 kg	No data available	Reduction in alcohol intake 9.2 g/week*	No data available	Increase in treatment 8.2%*

Explanation results: normal lettertype not significant, * $p < 0.05$, ** $p < 0.001$, between brackets (to) are the confidence intervals if available.
Abbreviations: DBP, diastolic blood pressure; DM, diabetes mellitus; FBG, fasting blood glucose; HT, hypertension; SBP, systolic blood pressure; WC, waist circumference; LTFU, lost to follow-up.

[a] Adjusted for age, sex, locality, body mass index.
[b] Adjusted for age, ethnicity and interactions.
[c] Adjustment for age.
[d] Adjusted for age, sex, clustering, baseline SBP.

Lara et al. 2008; Mohan et al. 2006; Nguyen et al. 2011; Onat et al. 2003; Salazar et al. 2005) and cross-sectional surveys (Dowse et al. 1995; Rossouw et al. 1993; Yu et al. 1999).

Blood pressure and hypertension

Nineteen studies measured the systolic blood pressure (SBP), and 15 of them included the diastolic blood pressure (DBP) as well, whereas 6 studies evaluated prevalence of hypertension. Except one (Lara et al. 2008), all studies showed significant reduction in blood pressure or hypertension prevalence. Reductions in mean systolic/diastolic ranged from 0.1/0.5 mmHg by worksite exercise breaks intervention (Lara et al. 2008) to 55.5/28.7 mmHg through introduction of a hypertension management structure with guidelines and training of staff (Nguyen et al. 2011). The majority of programmes with significantly decreased blood pressures contained health education, training of health care staff and introduction of guidelines.

Glucose, HB1Ac and diabetes

Four studies (Damião et al. 2010; Dowse et al. 1995; Harati et al. 2010; Kengne et al. 2009) evaluated fasting glucose levels, one study (Gill et al. 2008) evaluated HB1Ac and two (Khosravi et al. 2010; Ramachandran et al. 2006) evaluated absolute risk reduction in diabetes prevalence. Except one (Dowse et al. 1995), all the studies on glucose and HB1Ac found significant reductions in mean values. Ramachandran et al. (2006) found a significant reduction of 15.5% incidence of diabetes whilst Khosravi only found a meagre reduction of 0.8%. Most of the studies that had significant reduction were based on health education and training of health care staff with guidelines.

Weight, BMI, waist circumference

Less than half (7 out of 16 studies) found significant reductions in body sizes including in weight (Almeida-Pittito et al. 2010; Damião et al. 2010; Harati et al. 2010; Kengne et al. 2009), BMI (Gill et al. 2008; Lara et al. 2008; Rossouw et al. 1993), waist circumference (Damião et al. 2010; Harati et al. 2010; Krishnan et al. 2011) and prevalence of overweight (Krishnan et al. 2011). Two studies (Dowse et al. 1995; Gill et al. 2008) even showed an increase after the intervention in, respectively, prevalence of obesity and average BMI. Health programmes with a focus on physical activity and diet showed significant results.

Behaviour change (physical activity diet and smoking)

Seven out of 10 studies found a significant increase in physical activity, whereas two studies (Krishnan et al. 2011; Sarrafzadegan et al. 2009) showed a decrease in the follow-up. Most of the successful interventions to improve physical activity contained health education assisted by intensive training and coaching of exercises. Improved diets were shown through reduction of salt, fats, sugar and alcohol or increased intake of fruits and vegetables in 10 out of 13 studies mainly through health education interventions. Five out of nine studies showed a significant reduction in smoking, whereas one study showed an increase of intention to quit smoking (Kar et al. 2008). National and regional programmes with health promotion through media and health education showed to be effective interventions for smoking cessation.

Management and awareness of risk factors and retention of participants

Several studies showed a significant increase in knowledge of healthy lifestyle (Huang et al. 2011; Rossouw et al. 1993) in awareness of hypertension (Huang et al. 2011; Khosravi et al. 2010), treatment of hypertension (Chen, Wu, and Gu 2008; Huang et al. 2011; Khosravi et al. 2010; Salazar et al. 2005), control of hypertension and diabetes (Chen, Wu, and Gu 2008; Huang et al. 2011; Isaakidis et al. 2011; Jafar et al. 2009; Khosravi et al. 2010) and adherence (Kar et al. 2008; Ramachandran et al. 2006) after the intervention. Of the eight studies that measured retention of medium and high-risk patients for follow-up, only two (CSSS et al. 2007; Ramachandran et al. 2006) of them had at the end of the study more than 80% of the initial participants still in the study, and two were below 50% (Kengne et al. 2009; Onat et al. 2003). Studies that raised significantly levels of knowledge and behaviour contained intense health education through various methods (classes and print). Treatment and control of hypertension and diabetes increased mostly in studies where health care staff was rigorously trained, and adherence improved in studies where follow-up appointments were given with relatively short intervals and reminders were sent to patients.

Discussion

Several important insights have emerged from this systematic review of intervention studies to reduce the cardiovascular risk in LMICs. The reviewed studies were conducted on population level and on people with increased risk, and in urban as well as rural settings. There was a great variety of interventions with the four most prominent being: health promotion through media, health education, training health care staff and the implementation of guidelines for treatment. Additionally, some studies assessed adherence and cost-effectiveness of the interventions programmes.

Health education and health promotion through media

Several studies showed that health education in combination with other interventions have a significant impact on population with CVD health outcomes (Almeida-Pittito et al. 2010; Cappuccio et al. 2006; Chen, Wu, and Gu 2008). As a 2 mmHg reduction of blood pressure reduces death from strokes by 10%, it seems that these kinds of community interventions have a substantial public health benefit (Ford et al. 2007; Lewington et al. 2002). On a patient level, Jafar et al. (2009) showed that a combination of health education towards patients' households and training of general practitioners on management of hypertension has a strong impact on several important outcomes such as control of hypertension and reduction of mean blood pressure.

Other studies have also demonstrated a significant impact of health education on biomedical measurements such as HbA1c (Gill et al. 2008; Ramachandran et al.

2006). Huang et al. (2011) demonstrated an improvement in knowledge, behaviour and control of hypertension after an intervention of health education and training of health care providers. Knowledge on effects of risk factors and treatment approach more than doubled after the intervention. This might have resulted in significant reductions in salt and fatty products intake, pickled food and alcohol consumption as well as an increase in participation in physical exercise and increase in awareness, treatment and control of hypertension (Huang et al. 2011).

Similar to the results of the North Karelia study, the most significant lifestyle change in the current review was diet (Vartiainen et al. 1994) with more than three-quarters of the studies showing significant improvements.

The Isfahan Healthy Heart Programme shows that in case of diet, the best results were seen in the change of using non-hydrogenated instead of hydrogenated oils and the reduction of salt intake (Kelishadi et al. 2011). Although diet is the most significant lifestyle change this is often not reflected in reduction of weight or waist circumference. Overweight and obesity seem to be the most challenging risk factors and as most of the studies showed no significant reduction.

There are promising results from the CSSS group (2007) and Cappuccio's (2006) study on salt reduction and substitution in LMICs. The high salt intake in these settings is caused by personal use, in contrast to high salt intake due to consumption of processed foods in high-income countries (WHO 2002).

Training of health care providers and implementation of treatment guidelines

Various studies described the importance of intensive training of health care providers as the level of knowledge can be quite low in several health care settings (Fuster and Kelly 2010; Jafar et al. 2005). The studies that included training of health care providers in this review showed significant reductions in cardiovascular risk factors. Specifically in the studies that included task shifting, the training and supervision of health care providers were found to be essential. This review indicates that there are some promising results on task shifting of management of CVD risk factors from doctors to nurses (Gill et al. 2008; Kengne et al. 2009). These have been supported by clear supervision and the development of guidelines. Implementing existing guidelines (Kar et al. 2008) or designing them for the specific location (Gill et al. 2008) also showed good results in the review. In the Cochrane study (Fahey, Schroeder, and Ebrahim 2010) on interventions on hypertension control it is stated that there is a benefit if community-based clinics have an organised system of regular follow-up and that medication should be given by means of a stepped care approach by implementing a structured guideline.

It is useful to link these trainings to a recognised medical organisation that gives the training better content and professional esteem. It is important to look not only for improvement at the public system, but also private practices as studies show that sometimes even more than half of the patients with cardiovascular risk factors visit the private sector in LMICs (Kar et al. 2008). This review also shows that there is effective reduction of risk factors outside the health system, like on the worksite (Chen, Wu, and Gu 2008; Lara et al. 2008).

The Cuban example shows that even in LMICs there can be high success rates of treatment and control of hypertension if there is a focus on primary health care, and that medication is easily available and affordable (Orduñez-Garcia et al. 2006).

Follow-up and adherence

Follow-up and adherence remain key challenges in reduction of cardiovascular risk. Specifically, studies from sub-Saharan Africa still have high rates of drop out like Kengne et al. (2009) in this review or smaller studies like Labhardt et al. (2011) and Bovet et al. (2008). In all these studies the biggest loss to follow-up was in the first three months after diagnosis and after community screening. Bovet argued that it is important to have a structured follow-up after diagnosing hypertension as the majority of the patients (66%) failed to contact a clinic after the measurements. About 40% of these people stated that the main reason was that they lacked any symptoms, and about 15% mentioned treatment costs as barrier to adherence. Among the people that had visited a clinic, less than 10% were taking medication at the end of the year (Bovet et al. 2008).

One of the successes of the study of Kar et al. (2008) might be due to the fact that they follow the patients closely in the first few months with scheduled visits at the clinic at first, third and fifth months, which is more often than most standard treatment guidelines recommend. The adherence increased from 35% to 61% and the blood pressure decreased by 8 mmHg in the intervention group. Stricter follow-up schedules may, however, worsen the strain on the already stretched health systems in LMICs. Kar et al. (2008), however, showed in the feasibility part of their study, that this intensive management of CVD might be integrated in the general health system. It took 13.6 minutes per person to do a risk assessment and they calculated that it is feasible to integrate screening in the package of the health care worker. Kar et al. (2008) demonstrated in the same study that there is a connection between availability of medication and adherence. As the availability of medication dropped at the public health facility, so did the adherence rate.

Some studies show that interventions are much more effective among older people who seem to be more adherent than younger people (Bovet et al. 2008; Khosravi et al. 2010). The studies also show that the patients who tend to be more adherent are often highly educated, believe in the medication and have the support from their family (Jafar et al. 2009). Also co-morbidity with diabetes show better results for follow-up (Isaakidis et al. 2011). In Isaakidis et al.'s (2011) study the adherence of HIV medication in the same clinic was 15 times higher than antihypertensive adherence, possibly due to inequality of care as HIV patients received free health care, money for transportation, food and social support, whereas the hypertension patients got nothing.

Feasibility

Some community studies such as the national programme in Mauritius and the regional programmes in Iran, Indonesia, India, China and South Africa have demonstrated significant reductions in cardiovascular risk factors (Dowse et al. 1995; Khosravi et al. 2010; Krishnan et al. 2011; Mohan et al. 2006; Rossouw et al. 1993; Sarrafzadegan et al. 2009; Yu et al. 1999). These studies have shown the effectiveness of comprehensive programmes in LMICs. The greatest challenge remains the political willingness of local authorities and the availability of resources to replicate and maintain support such programmes in other LMICs. The initial programmes have been supported to a large extent by WHO (Dowse et al. 1995; Krishnan et al.

2011; Sarrafzadegan et al. 2009). Because of relatively high costs and intensive support these programmes might be challenging to sustain or scale up. Only a few studies have included in their study the costs (Jafar et al. 2011; Ramachandran et al. 2007) and feasibility (Kar et al. 2008). The study of Jafar et al. (2011) showed that a combination of patient education and training of general practitioners was the most cost-effective with 23 US dollars (USD) per 1.0 mmHg reduction in blood pressure among hypertensive patients. They measured the annual costs of their intervention at 3.99 USD per patient. Ramachandran et al. (2006) came to the conclusion that medication and lifestyle advices are cost-effective interventions for preventing diabetes among high risk individuals.

As almost one billion people live today in urban slums and they are particularly at risk for CVDs, it was striking that there were no large population studies from these settings. The same counts for the close to a billion people from Africa where only 5 of the 26 studies were taking place. In the light of the fact that the urban population of Sub-Saharan Africa is predicted to triple in the next 30 years (UN-HABITAT 2010), there is a strong need to develop prevention programmes for those people at risk, and specifically for the slum-dwellers who will continue to form the majority of urban populations on this continent.

Limitations

Literature reviews are prone to publication bias (Wright et al. 2007) and it is likely that studies with inconclusive or negative results might have been overlooked by publishers. Although we set a minimum of one year of follow-up this is still a short period of time, which makes it difficult to generalise the outcomes to longer term periods.

As most of the studies have implemented a variety of interventions, it is difficult to determine which part of the intervention has been essential for the reduction of the cardiovascular risk factors. In order to understand the interaction between different parts of the intervention and the success of elements inside the intervention there should be more focus on process evaluation. Only one study (Kar et al. 2008) has elements of process evaluation by showing percentages of patients where the drugs were prescribed according to the protocol and measurements as per guideline were done.

The Isfahan study published a separate article on the process evaluation of the study, which gives more insight into the functioning of their intervention (Rabiei et al. 2009).

Less than half of the studies used a control group which makes it difficult to separate the outcomes from possible secular trend. Some studies (Harati et al. 2010) with control group show that interventions on BMI or waist circumference have only a modest difference before and after the implementation of the programme but a significant difference with the control group. The main reason given for this finding according to the authors was the strong secular trend of rising rates of overweight and obesity. The rise of obesity vs reduction on other risk factors in the national programme in Mauritius shows how difficult it is to break this global trend.

Although we have tried to restrict our review to LMICs it is evident that there is still a great heterogeneity in the settings of these studies. For example, there is a big difference between a white South-African community (Rossouw et al. 1993) and a rural Cambodian community (Isaakidis et al. 2011).

Additionally, because of limited resources, we restricted our literature search to only papers published in English. It is possible that the results of studies published in non-English languages may differ, which might affect our study conclusions. Furthermore, as the level of awareness and knowledge about CVD risk factors is still very low in LMICs it is easier to achieve positive findings on interventions with health education and health promotion through media (Gaziano, Galea, and Reddy 2007). This means that the effect of some interventions in this review might be reduced in the future when these countries develop and awareness will rise, but for now there is still a lot to gain.

Key messages

(1) There have been effective community-based programmes to reduce cardio-vascular risk factors in LMICs but they are very limited, specifically to the urban poor.
(2) A key element of the intervention should be introducing treatment guidelines and training of health care providers.
(3) Health education for population and patients at risk with focus on diet and salt reduction is also showing good results.
(4) Combining several interventions, with an intensive follow-up schedule and a community-sensitive approach, that can be sustainable and scalable for LMICs are urgently required.

Acknowledgements

S.vd.V and S.O. receive funding from the AMC Foundation. We thank Dr Gabriela Gomez, Dr Lizzy Brewster, Dr Constance Schultsz and Dr Remare Ettare for their useful comments on this review.

References

Addo, J., L. Smeeth, and D. A. Leon. 2007. "Hypertension in Sub-saharan Africa: A Systematic Review." *Hypertension* 50 (6): 1012–1018.

Agyemang, C. 2006. "Rural and Urban Differences in Blood Pressure and Hypertension in Ghana, West Africa." *Public Health* 120 (6): 525–533.

Almeida-Pittito, B., A. T. Hirai, D. S. Sartorelli, S. G. Gimeno, S. R. Ferreira, and Japanese–Brazilian Diabetes Study Group. 2010. "Impact of a 2-Year Intervention Program on Cardiometabolic Profile According to the Number of Goals Achieved." *Brazilian Journal of Medical and Biological Research* 43 (11): 1088–1094.

Bhalla, V., C. W. Fong, S. K. Chew, and K. Satku. 2006. "Changes in the Levels of Major Cardiovascular Risk Factors in the Multi-Ethnic Population in Singapore after 12 Years of a National Non-communicable Disease Intervention Programme." *Singapore Medical Journal* 47: 841–850.

Bovet, P., J. P. Gervasoni, M. Mkamba, M. Balampama, C. Lengeler, and F. Paccaud. 2008. "Low Utilization of Health Care Services Following Screening for Hypertension in Dar Es Salaam (Tanzania): A Prospective Population-Based Study." *BMC Public Health* 16 (8): 407.

Cappuccio, F. P., S. M. Kerry, F. B. Micah, J. Plange-Rhule, and J. B. Eastwood. 2006. "A Community Programme to Reduce Salt Intake and Blood Pressure in Ghana." *Public Health* 24: 6–13.

Chen, J., X. Wu, and D. Gu. 2008. "Hypertension and Cardiovascular Diseases Intervention in the Capital Steel and Iron Company and Beijing Fangshan Community." *Obesity Review* 9 (Suppl. 1): 142–145.

China Salt Substitute Study Collaborative Group (CSSS). 2007. "Salt Substitution: A Low-Cost Strategy for Blood Pressure Control among Rural Chinese. A Randomized, Controlled Trial." *Journal of Hypertension* 25 (10), 2011–2018.

Damião, R., D. S. Sartorelli, A. Hirai, F. Massimino, J. Poletto, M. R. Bevilacqua, R. Chaim, et al. 2010. "Nutritional Intervention Programme among a Japanese-Brazilian Community: Procedures and Results According to Gender." *Public Health Nutrition* 13 (9): 1453–1461.

Dowse, G. K., H. Gareeboo, K. G. Alberti, P. Zimmet, J. Tuomilehto, A. Purran, D. Fareed, P. Chitson, and V. R. Collins. 1995. "Changes in Population Cholesterol Concentrations and Other Cardiovascular Risk Factor Levels after Five Years of the Non-Communicable Disease Intervention Programme in Mauritius." *British Medical Journal* 311: 1255–1259.

Fahey, T., K. Schroeder, and S. Ebrahim. 2010. "Interventions Used to Improve Control of Blood Pressure in Patients with Hypertension." *Cochrane Database System Review* 3: CD005182.

Ford, E. S., U. A. Ajani, J. B. Croft, J. A. Critchley, D. R. Labarthe, and T. E. Kottke. 2007. "Explaining the Decrease in US Deaths from Coronary Disease, 1980–2000." *New England Journal Medicine* 356: 2388–2398.

Fuentes, R., N. Ilmaniemi, E. Laurikainen, J. Tuomilehto, and A. Nissinen. 2000. "Hypertension in Developing Economies: A Review of Population-Based Studies Carried Out from 1980 to 1998." *Journal of Hypertension* 18 (5): 521–529.

Fuster, V., and B. B. Kelly. 2010. *Promoting Cardiovascular Health in the Developing World.* Washington, DC: National Academies Press.

Gaziano, T. A., G. Galea, and K. S. Reddy. 2007. "Scaling Up Interventions for Chronic Disease Prevention: The Evidence." *Lancet* 370 (9603): 1939–1946.

Gill, G. V., C. Price, D. Shandu, M. Dedicoat, and D. Wilkinson. 2008. "An Effective System of Nurse-Led Diabetes Care in Rural Africa." *Diabetes Medicine* 25 (5): 606–611.

Godfrey, R., and M. Julien. 2005. "Urbanisation and Health." *Clinical Medicine* 5 (2): 137–141.

Harati, H., F. Hadaegh, A. A. Momenan, L. Ghanei, M. R. Bozorgmanesh, A. Ghanbarian, P. Mirmiran, and F. Azizi. 2010. "Reduction in Incidence of Type 2 Diabetes by Lifestyle Intervention in a Middle Eastern Community." *American Journal Preventive Medicine* 38 (6): 628–636.

Huang, S., X. Hu, H. Chen, D. Xie, X. Gan, Y. Wu, S. Nie, and J. Wu. 2011. "The Positive Effect of an Intervention Program on the Hypertension Knowledge and Lifestyles of Rural Residents over the Age of 35 Years in an Area of China." *Hypertension Research* 34 (4): 503–508.

Isaakidis, P., M. E. Raguenaud, C. Say, H. De Clerck, C. Khim, R. Pottier, S. Kuoch, et al. 2011. "Treatment of Hypertension in Rural Cambodia: Results from a 6-Year Programme." *Journal Human Hypertension* 25 (4): 241–249.

Jafar, T. H., J. Hatcher, N. Poulter, M. Islam, S. Hashmi, Z. Qadri, R. Bux, et al. 2009. "Community-based Interventions to Promote Blood Pressure Control in a Developing Country: A Cluster Randomized Trial." *Annals Internal Medicine* 151: 593–601.

Jafar, T. H., M. Islam, R. Bux, N. Poulter, J. Hatcher, N. Chaturvedi, S. Ebrahim, and P. Cosgrove, and Hypertension Research Group. 2011. Cost-effectiveness of Community-based Strategies for Blood Pressure Control in a Low-income Developing Country: Findings from a Cluster-Randomized, Factorial-controlled Trial." *Circulation* 124 (15): 1615–1625.

Jafar, T. H., S. Jessani, F. H. Jafary, M. Ishaq, R. Orakzai, S. Orakzai, A.S. Levey, and N. Chaturvedi. 2005. "General Practitioners' Approach to Hypertension in Urban Pakistan: Disturbing Trends in Practice." *Circulation* 111: 1278–1283.

Kar, S. S., J. S. Thakur, S. Jain, and R. Kumar. 2008. "Cardiovascular Disease Risk Management in a Primary Health Care Setting of North India." *Indian Heart Journal* 60 (1): 19–25.

Kelishadi, R., N. Sarrafzadegan, G. H. Sadri, R. Pashmi, N. Mohammadifard, A. A. Tavasoli, A. Amani, K. Rabiei, A. Khosravi, and A. Bahonar. 2011. "Short-term Results of a Community-based Program on Promoting Healthy Lifestyle for Prevention and Control of Chronic Diseases in a Developing Country Setting: Isfahan Healthy Heart Program." *Asia-Pacific Journal of Public Health* 23 (4): 518–533.

Kengne, A. P., P. K. Awah, L. L. Fezeu, E. Sobngwi, and J. C. Mbanya. 2009. "Primary Health Care for Hypertension by Nurses in Rural and Urban Sub-Saharan Africa." *Journal of Clinical Hypertension* 11 (10): 564–572.

Khosravi, A., G. K. Mehr, R. Kelishadi, S. Shirani, M. A. Tavassoli, F. Noori, and N. Sarrafzadegan. 2010. "The Impact of a 6-Year Comprehensive Community Trial on the Awareness, Treatment and Control Rates of Hypertension in Iran: Experiences from the Isfahan Healthy Heart Program." *BMC Cardiovascular Disorders* 21: 10–61.

Krishnan, A., R. Ekowati, N. Baridalyne, N. Kusumawardani, S. K. Suhardi Kapoor, and J. Leowski. 2011. "Evaluation of Community-based Interventions for Non-communicable Diseases: Experiences from India and Indonesia." *Health Promotion International* 26 (3): 276–289.

Labhardt, N. D., J. R. Balo, M. Ndam, E. Manga, and B. Stoll. 2011. "Improved Retention Rates with Low-Cost Interventions in Hypertension and Diabetes Management in a Rural African Environment of Nurse-Led Care: A Cluster-Randomised Trial." *Tropical Medicine International Health*, 6. doi:10.1111/j.1365-3156.2011.02827.x. [Epub ahead of print]

Lara, A., A. K. Yancey, R. Tapia-Conye, Y. Flores, P. Kuri-Morales, R. Mistry, E. Subirats, and W. J. McCarthy. 2008. "Pausa Para tu Salud: Reduction of Weight and Waistlines by Integrating Exercise Breaks into Workplace Organizational Routine." *Prevention Chronic Diseases* 5 (1): A12.

Lewington, S., R. Clarke, N. Qizilbash, R. Peto, and R. Collins. 2002. "Age-specific Relevance of Usual Blood Pressure to Vascular Mortality: A Metaanalysis of Individual Data for One Million Adults in 61 Prospective Studies." *Lancet* 360: 1903–1913.

Lopez, A. D., C. D. Mathers, M. Ezzati, D. T. Jamison, and C. J. Murray. 2006. "Global and Regional Burden of Disease and Risk Factors, 2001: Systematic Analysis of Population Health Data." *Lancet* 367: 1747–1757.

Mohan, V., C. S. Shanthirani, M. Deepa, M. Datta, O. D. Williams, and R. Deepa. 2006. "Community Empowerment – A Successful Model for Prevention of Non-communicable Diseases in India. The Chennai Urban Population Study (CUPS –17)." *Journal of Association of Physicians of India* 54: 858–862.

Moher, D., A. Liberati, J. Tetzlaff, D. G. Altman, and PRISMA Group. 2009. "Preferred Reporting Items for Systematic Reviews and Meta-Analyses: The PRISMA Statement." *PLoS Medicine* 6 (7).

Nguyen, Q. N., S. T. Pham, V. L. Nguyen, S. Wall, L. Weinehall, R. Bonita, and P. Byass. 2011. "Implementing a Hypertension Management Programme in a Rural Area: Local Approaches and Experiences from Ba-Vi District, Vietnam." *BMC Public Health* 17 (11): 325.

Onat, A., I. Soydan, L. Tokgözoğlu, V. Sansoy, N. Koylan, N. Domaniç, D. Ural, and Riskburden Study Group, Turkish Society of Cardiology. 2003. "Guideline Implementation in a Multicenter Study with an Estimated 44% Relative Cardiovascular Event Risk Reduction." *Clinical Cardiology* 26 (5): 243–249.

Orduñez-Garcia, P., J. L. Munoz, D. Pedraza, A. Espinosa-Brito, L. C. Silva, and R. S. Cooper. 2006. "Success in Control of Hypertension in a Low Resource Setting: The Cuban Experience." *Journal of Hypertension* 24: 845–849.

Pearson, T. A., T. L. Bazzarre, S. R. Daniels, J. M. Fair, S. P. Fortmann, B. A. Franklin, L. B. Goldstein, et al. 2003. "American Heart Association Guide for Improving Cardiovascular Health at the Community Level: A Statement for Public Health Practitioners, Healthcare Providers, and Health Policy Makers from the American Heart Association Expert Panel on Population and Prevention Science." *Circulation* 107 (4): 645–651.

Puska, P., J. T. Salonen, and A. Nissinen. 1983. "Change in Risk Factors for Coronary Heart Disease during 10 Years of a Community Intervention Programme (North Karelia Project)." *British Medical Journal* 7: 1840–1844.

Rabiei, K., R. Kelishadi, N. Sarrafzadegan, H. A. Abedi, M. Alavi, K. Heidari, A. Bahonar, M. Boshtam, K. Zare, and S. Sadeghi. 2009. "Process Evaluation of a Community-based Program for Prevention and Control of Non-communicable Disease in a Developing Country: The Isfahan Healthy Heart Program, Iran." *BMC Public Health* 12 (9): 57.

Ramachandran, A., C. Snehalatha, S. Mary, B. Mukesh, A. D. Bhaskar, V. Vijay, and Indian Diabetes Prevention Programme (IDPP). 2006. "The Indian Diabetes Prevention Programme Shows that Lifestyle Modification and Metformin Prevent Type 2 Diabetes in Asian Indian subjects with Impaired Glucose Tolerance (IDPP-1)." *Diabetologia* 49 (2): 289–297.

Ramachandran, A., C. Snehalatha, A. Yamuna, S. Mary, and Z. Ping. 2007. "Cost-effectiveness of the Interventions in the Primary Prevention of Diabetes among Asian Indians: Within-trial Results of the Indian Diabetes Prevention Programme (IDPP)." *Diabetes Care* 30 (10): 2548–2552.

Rossouw, J. E., P. L. Jooste, D. O. Chalton, E. R. Jordaan, M. L. Langenhoven, P. C. Jordaan, M. Steyn, A. S. Swanepoel, and L. J. Rossouw. 1993. "Community-based Intervention: The Coronary Risk Factor Study (CORIS)." *International Journal of Epidemiology* 22: 428–438.

Salazar, M. R., H. A. Carbajal, M. Aizpurúa, B. Riondet, H. F. Rodrigo, V. Rechifort, S. M. Quaini, and R. F. Echeverria. 2005. "Decrease of Blood Pressure by Community-based Strategies." *Medicina (B Aires)* 65 (6): 507–512.

Sarrafzadegan, N., R. Kelishadi, A. Esmaillzadeh, N. Mohammadifard, K. Rabiei, H. Roohafza, L. Azadbakht, et al. 2009. "Do Lifestyle Interventions Work in Developing Countries? Findings from the Isfahan Healthy Heart Program in the Islamic Republic of Iran." *Bulletin of World Health Organization* 87 (1): 39–50.

UN-HABITAT. 2010. *State of the African Cities 2010: Governance, Inequalities and Urban Land Markets.* Nairobi: UN-HABITAT.

Vartiainen, E., P. Puska, J. Pekkanen, J. Tuomilehto, and P. Jousilahti. 1994. "Changes in Risk Factors Explain Changes in Mortality from Ischaemic Heart Disease in Finland." *British Medical Journal* 309: 23–27.

Walker, R. W., D. G. McLarty, H. M. Kitange, D. Whiting, G. Masuki, D. M. Mtasiwa, H. Machibya, N. Unwin, and K. G. Alberti. 2000. "Stroke Mortality in Urban and Rural Tanzania. Adult Morbidity and Mortality Project." *Lancet* 355 (9216): 1684–1687.

WHO. 2002. *The World Health Report 2002: Reducing Risks, Promoting Healthy Life.* Geneva: World Health Organization.

WHO. 2005. *Preventing Chronic Diseases: A Vital Investment.* Geneva: World Health Organization.

WHO. 2007. *Prevention of Cardiovascular Disease: Guidelines for Assessment and Management of Total Cardiovascular Risk.* Geneva: World Health Organization.

WHO. 2011. *2008–2013 Action Plan for the Global Strategy for the Prevention and Control of Noncommunicable Diseases.* Geneva: World Health Organization. http://www.who.int/nmh/publications/ncd_action_plan_en.pdf

Wright, R. W., R. A. Brand, W. Dunn, and K. P. Spindler. 2007. "How to Write a Systematic Review." *Clinical Orthopaedics and Related Research* 455: 23–29.

Yu, Z., G. Song, Z. Guo, G. Zheng, H. Tian, E. Vartiainen, P. Puska, and A. Nissinen. 1999. "Changes in Blood Pressure, Body Mass Index, and Salt Consumption in a Chinese Population." *Preventive Medicine* 29 (3): 165–172.

Policy initiatives, culture and the prevention and control of chronic non-communicable diseases (NCDs) in the Caribbean

T. Alafia Samuels[a], Cornelia Guell[a], Branka Legetic[b] and Nigel Unwin[a]

[a]*Faculty of Medical Sciences, University of West Indies, Cave Hill Campus, Barbados;* [b]*Health Surveillance and Disease Management, Non Communicable Disease Project, Pan American Health Organization, Washington, DC, USA*

Objective. To explore interactions between disease burden, culture and the policy response to non-communicable diseases (NCDs) within the Caribbean, a region with some of the highest prevalence rates, morbidity and mortality from NCDs in the Americas.

Methods. We undertook a wide ranging narrative review, drawing on a variety of peer reviewed, government and intergovernmental literature.

Results. Although the Caribbean is highly diverse, linguistically and ethnically, it is possible to show how 'culture' at the macro-level has been shaped by shared historic, economic and political experiences and ties. We suggest four broad groupings of countries: the English-speaking Caribbean Community (CARICOM); the small island states that are still colonies or departments of colonial powers; three large-Spanish speaking countries; and Haiti, which although part of CARICOM is culturally distinct. We explore how NCD health policies in the region stem from and are influenced by the broad characteristics of these groupings, albeit played out in varied ways in individual countries. For example, the Port of Spain declaration (2007) on NCDs can be understood as the product of the co-operative and collaborative relationships with CARICOM, which are based on a shared broad culture. We note, however, that studies investigating the relationships between the formation of NCD policy and culture (at any level) are scarce.

Conclusion. Within the Caribbean region it is possible to discern relationships between culture at the macro-level and the formation of NCD policy. However, there is little work that directly assesses the interactions between culture and NCD policy formation. The Caribbean with its cultural diversity and high burden of NCDs provides an ideal environment within which to undertake further studies to better understand the interactions between culture and health policy formation.

Introduction

Chronic non-communicable diseases (NCDs) are the major cause of mortality and morbidity in the world as a whole, and in all countries apart from the very poorest (World Health Organization 2008). It is increasingly recognised that public policy has a major role to play in the prevention and control of NCDs, with the UN High Level meeting on NCDs in September 2011, for example, agreeing on the need for population-wide interventions that employ education, legislative, regulatory and fiscal measures (World Health Organization 2011).

The countries within the Caribbean region have some of the highest NCD morbidity and mortality rates in the Americas, and over the past few years many of them have been very active in drawing up policy responses to this growing NCD epidemic. The Caribbean is culturally highly diverse. In this paper we explore interactions between disease burden, culture and the policy response to NCDs within the Caribbean. First we lay the scene by describing the countries and their disease burden, and then consider culture, and the experiences that have shaped it across the region. We go on to examine the experience to date of developing and implementing policy initiatives and how those relate to the cultural milieus within the Caribbean.

The Caribbean countries and NCDs

The Caribbean countries

The Caribbean population of 43 million across 28 countries (Figure 1; Table 1) exhibits a wide range of economic and social conditions. There are 10 high-income countries, of which Barbados is the only one that is also classified as 'developed' on

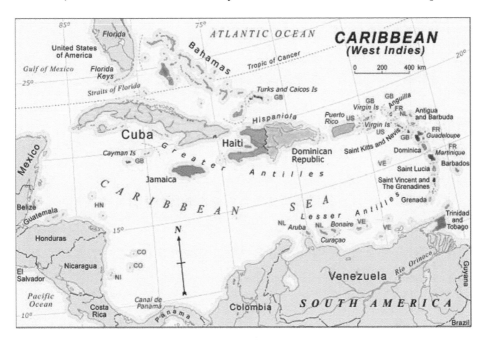

Figure 1. Map of the Caribbean.
Note: NB Suriname, not shown, is the next country to the south east of Guyana.
Source: The Atlas of Canada, Caribbean, http://atlas.nrcan.gc.ca/site/english/maps/reference/international/caribbean. Reproduced with the permission of Natural Resources Canada 2012, courtesy of the Atlas of Canada.

Table 1. Selected demographic, economic and population health characteristics of Caribbean countries and territories.

CARICOM member countries	Popula-tion (1000s)	% < 15 years	% ≥60 years	Total fertility rate[a]	Life expectancy at birth	System of government (year of independence)	Gross national income 2010 US$ per capita[b]
						All independent CARICOM countries are multi-party parliamentary democracies	
Anguilla[c]	15	24	11	1.8	80.8	UKOT	14,009
Antigua and Barbuda	87	26	10	2.1	75.3	(1981)	11,856
Bahamas	343	22.5	10.4	1.9	75.4	(1973)	21,663
Barbados	286	19	13	1.7	74.1	(1966)	13,393
Belize	312	35	5.7	2.8	75.9	(1981)	3939
Bermuda[c]	68	18	20	2	80.6	UKOT	115,176[e]
Cayman Islands[c]	50	19	14	1.9	80.6	UKOT	51,677
Dominica	73	23	13	2.1	75.8	(1978)	6673
Grenada	108	25	12	2.2	72.8	(1974)	6883
Guyana	754	33.6	6.4	2.2	69.7	(1966)	2952
Haiti	9993	35.9	6.5	3.3	61.9	(1804)	612
Jamaica	2741	29.1	10.6	2.3	73	(1962)	4653
Montserrat	5	27	9	1.3	72.9	UKOT	8623
Saint Kitts and Nevis	50	23	10	1.8	74.4	(1983)	9858
Saint Lucia	161	23	12	1.8	76.7	(1979)	5486
Saint Vincent and Grenadines	104	25	10	1.9	73.9	(1979)	6323
Suriname	525	28.6	9.3	2.3	70.4	(1975)	7047
Trinidad and Tobago	1341	20.6	10.6	1.6	70	(1962)	15,641
Turks and Caicos Islands[c]	43	23	5	1.7	79	UKOT	39,391
Virgin Islands (UK)[c]	25	18	10	1.7	77.5	UKOT	–
Dutch Caribbean							

Table 1 (*Continued*)

	Popula-tion (1000s)	% < 15 years	% ≥60 years	Total fertility rate[a]	Life expectancy at birth	System of government (year of independence)	Gross national income 2010 US$ per capita[b]
Aruba[d]	105	18	16	1.9	75.5	Full internal self-government (1986)	21,476
Netherlands Antilles	229	–	–	2	76.9	Dependents of Netherlands	20,108
Latin Caribbean							
Cuba	11,258	17.3	16.9	1.5	79	Centrally planned economy since 1959 (1898)	5621
The Dominican Republic[d]	9927	31	8.9	2.6	73.3	Multi-party representative democracy (1844)	4952
Puerto Rico[d]	3749	21	18	1.8	79.1	Self-governing commonwealth in association with the USA	17,433
French Caribbean							
Guadeloupe	461	22.5	17.1	2.1	79.7	Overseas department of France	–
Martinique	406	19.4	19.9	1.9	80.4	Overseas department of France	–
US Caribbean							
Virgin Islands (US)	110	–	–	1.8	79.2	Unincorporated territory of the USA	–

[a]Births per woman.
[b]Gross National Income per capita in US dollars (Source of data: UN data).
United Nations Statistical Division: National Accounts Main Aggregates Database http://unstats.un.org/unsd/snaama/dnllist.asp
Demographic data from PAHO Basic Indicators
[c]CARICOM associate members.
[d]CARICOM observers.
[e]Bermuda has the third highest per capita GNI in the world based on offshore financial services and high-end tourism experience, with over 500,000 visitors each year and a small population.
Other CARICOM observers are Curacao, St Maarten, Colombia, Venezuela and Mexico.
UKOT (United Kingdom Overseas Territory), crown colonies with limited internal self-government.

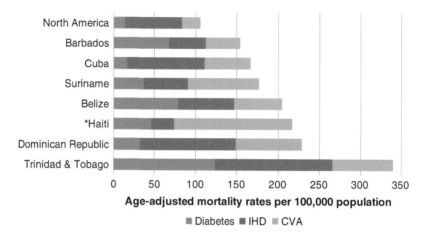

Figure 2. Age-adjusted mortality rates per 100,000 population for diabetes, Ischemic Heart disease and cerebrovascular disease in select Caribbean countries 2010.
Source: PAHO (2012); *Haiti-PAHO (2008) data.

the UN Human Development Index, through to low-income Haiti with a level of development similar to Papua New Guinea or Yemen. Among the remaining countries, the majority (14) are upper middle-income countries, and two, Guyana and Belize, are low middle income. Cuba's health status is equivalent to that of high-income countries.

In all states, besides Cuba, liberal democracy is the norm, with elections leading to the peaceful transfer of political power, and there is dynamic entrepreneurship and a significant middle-class. The varied political economies, histories of labour movements and social welfare systems in the Caribbean countries have produced significant socio-economic disparity (World Bank 2002) both between and within countries.

The epidemiological transition

With the exception of Haiti, the Caribbean countries have completed the epidemiological and demographic transition, with rapidly ageing populations (see Table 1 for proportion of the population ≥60 years). In a little over half of all countries fertility rates are below replacement levels (Table 1). Ageing of the population, successes in primary health care, economic development and increasingly unhealthy behaviours, for example indicated by high levels of obesity in many countries (Henry 2004), are helping to fuel the epidemiological transition.

The median life expectancy of men in the Caribbean is 5.5 years (range 2.4–7.9) shorter than that of women (Pan American Health Organization 2010), which has been suggested to be attributed to socially determined gender roles associated with higher rates of tobacco and alcohol use and abuse among men (Wilks *et al.* 2007/8, CAREC 2010a, 2010b, 2011, In Press), higher rates of HIV/AIDS and injuries (Pan American Health Organization 2010), as well as the poor utilisation of health services by men (Brenzel *et al.* 2001).

NCD morbidity and mortality

NCDs account for 75% of all deaths in the region of the Americas, with the Caribbean having the highest proportional NCD mortality rates (Pan American Health Organization 2010). Approximately 30% of all deaths are premature (occur before the age of 70), preventable NCD deaths (Alwan 2010), thus contributing to lost productivity and escalating health care costs (CARICOM 2007b).

In Trinidad and Tobago, Suriname and Guyana, people of South Asian origin are at a higher risk than African origin populations of ischaemic heart disease and diabetes (Miller *et al.* 1996). Diabetes mortality in Trinidad and Tobago is 600% higher than in North America (USA and Canada), and cardiovascular disease mortality in Trinidad and Tobago, Guyana and Suriname is 84%, 62% and 56% higher, respectively, than in North America (Pan American Health Organization 2010) (Figure 2).

In Barbados the incidence and associated mortality from diabetes-related lower extremity amputations are among the highest recorded in the world (Hennis *et al.* 2004, Hambleton *et al.* 2009). Overall Haiti has the highest stroke mortality, and Trinidad and Tobago, the highest diabetes-associated mortality in the Caribbean.

Chronic NCDs account for >90% of all deaths in Cuba, due in part to ageing of the population, low levels of injury and the successful prevention and control of communicable diseases. The most important risk factor for NCDs in Cuba is tobacco use, which is 43% among males and 29% among females (World Health Organization 2009). In 2007, tobacco smoking accounted for 86% of lung cancers, 78% of chronic obstructive pulmonary disease, 28% of ischaemic heart disease and 26% of cerebrovascular disease (Varona *et al.* 2009).

The wide range of mortality rates between countries is associated with the economic diversity of the region and the ethnic mix of the countries. Those countries with large East Indian/South Asian populations have correspondingly high diabetes

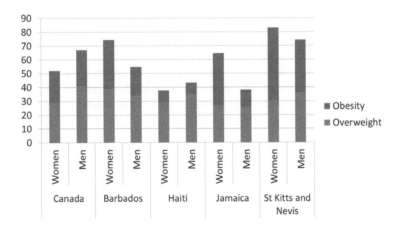

Figure 3. Prevalence (%) of overweight and obesity in selected countries.
Source: World Health Organization (2012) Global data base on Body Mass Index: Canada (2004); Cuba (2002); Guyana (2000); Haiti (2006); CAREC (2010b); Wilks et al. 2007/8; CAREC (2011).

prevalence and mortality. High-income countries like Barbados and Trinidad and Tobago, with these levels of disposable income, and market penetration of high-fat fast food outlets, have correspondingly high rates of obesity, diabetes and heart disease and stroke, while the middle-income islands in general have lower rates. However, the historically determined, shared dietary preference for high salt foods also contributes to high rates of hypertension, heart disease and stroke.

Prevalence of major NCD risk factors

Smoking

In general the prevalence of tobacco smoking is relatively low in the Caribbean, at 3% for women and 11% for men (CAREC 2010a, 2010b, 2011, In Press). Smoking rates among children 13–15 years are higher than among adults, at 5–11% (The Global Youth Tobacco Survey Collaborative Group 2002). Marijuana is illegal, but is widely used, and may account, in part, for the relatively low rates of tobacco use.

Overweight and obesity

Overweight and obesity are highly prevalent in the Caribbean, and higher in women than in men (Figure 3), which may reflect a greater cultural acceptance of obesity in women. As the region has become more developed, sedentary lifestyles are now the norm (Henry 2004). Fast foods are ubiquitous. While some international fast food chains, especially those providing a variety of chicken dishes, can be found in almost every Caribbean country, local fast food chains as well as street food vending are equally popular. Marketing of sugary sweet drinks is unrelenting. There is evidence that poorer families make greater use of fast foods than wealthier as a relatively economic way of feeding their families (Henry 2004), and with increasing economic austerity this is likely to increase.

Physical inactivity

Among children between the ages of 13 and 15 years in six Caribbean countries, 36–57% sit for more than three hours of leisure time each day mostly playing computer games (CDC n.d.). In the adult population, prevalence of low physical activity ranges between 59% in Barbados (CAREC In Press) and 34.6% in Dominica (CAREC 2011). Physical inactivity increased in Jamaican adults from 17.4% in 2000 to 29.5% in 2008 (Wilks et al. 2007/8).

Alcohol

Alcohol abuse is significant. Historically the Caribbean economy was based on sugar cane production, but since advent of the European Union closed that market, there has been an increasing emphasis on the use of sugar to produce rum. Alcohol use among men, even to excess, is socially acceptable in the region (Pyne et al. 2002). Alcohol is the leading cause of morbidity in this region through its impact on cardiovascular disease, injuries and violence and neuropsychiatric disorders (Rehm et al. 2006). STEPS NCD risk factor data from four CARICOM countries indicate levels of problem drinking among men (five or more drinks on any one day in the past week), ranging from 9.2% to 27.7% (CAREC 2010a, 2010b, 2011, In Press).

Shared histories and cultures

Defining 'culture'

To refer to 'culture' in the Caribbean context – and elsewhere – is a problematic endeavour. Definitions of culture include 'the language and accumulated knowledge, beliefs, practices, assumptions and values that are passed between individuals, groups and generations (Eckersley 2007, p. 194), or more specifically 'areas such as language, the imaginative, visual and performing arts, music, patterns of eating, and images such as dress and conceptions of beauty' which provide 'clues into the set of norms, beliefs and values that form the culture' (Burton 2009, p. 4). From an anthropological perspective, 'culture' is a complex and multifaceted concept, locally, politically, economically influenced and variably distributed between generations and population groups. We aim to follow the latter and consider 'culture' in its widest possible remit, as commonalities that shape and is shaped by shared historic and political-economic experiences. More precisely, our approach to 'cultural responses to NCDs' in this paper conceives of 'culture' in this macroview of shared histories and experiences that create commonalities and cooperation within the region.

Shared history and ethnicities

The Caribbean countries share a common history from colonialism, plantation slavery and indentureship towards emancipation and nation-building (Beckles and Shepherd 2006). Much political independence has been achieved in the region (with the exception of micro-island states, still reliant on colonial powers, and Puerto Rico, which remains in association with the USA). However, economic independence seems less established. Caribbean economies still partially rely on external sources for loans and investment. This reliance has been shaped by the political agendas of the cold war to present day international trade interests of Europe, the USA (Beckles and Shepherd 2006) and increasingly new economic powers such as China. Within countries, the remnants of the white plantation economy are still evident in the concentration of wealth among their descendants.

Ethnicity is related to the colonial history of the region. There are few indigenous populations remaining in the region (Montenegro and Stephens 2006), mostly Maya in the mainland countries of Guyana, Suriname and Belize, and Kalinago in the mainland and Lesser Antilles such as Dominica (Beckles and Shepherd 2006). Descendants of the African slave trade comprise the vast majority of the population. Trinidad and Tobago and Guyana have both approximately 50% South Asian (referred to as 'East Indian' in the Caribbean) populations from indentured labourers, with large migrations occurring in the nineteenth century as part of replacing slave labour following abolition. There is a rich ethnic mix in most countries, with descendants from Africa (for example ethnic groups from Ghana, Nigeria and Senegal), Asia (South Asian and smaller Chinese populations) and Europe (UK, France, Spain, Netherlands and Portugal), and high rates of inter-marriage in most Caribbean countries (Beckles and Shepherd 2006). Although much less important than only 40–50 years ago, when many countries were gaining independence from colonial masters, social and economic hierarchies based on colour and ethnicity are still highly apparent in many Caribbean countries. Wealth tends to be disproportionately concentrated in white and lighter skinned groups, reflecting in part descendants of the plantocracy and the legacy of racism that gave greater opportunities to lighter skinned people. In some countries, notably Trinidad and Tobago and Guyana, politics in the past have divided along ethnic group lines, with East Indians and Africans supporting different political parties. Although less clear-cut today than at independence, some of this persists.

Gender and family structure

Family structure in the Caribbean is often described as matrifocal and is studied widely for its great diversity in domestic relations and gender roles (Barrow 1996). Regional gender studies investigate Caribbean women's dominant care-giving roles in the light of the power relations that underlie absent fathers, single or mother–grandmother households and common law unions (Barrow 1996), and rapidly changing gender roles in the Caribbean (Barriteau 2003). Shaped by the legacy of slavery and later labour migration, 24% (in Belize) to 59% (in Saint Lucia) of households are female-led (United Nations 2010), and women's participation in the labour force is common, with non-agricultural participation ranging from 34% in Suriname to 47% in Barbados (World Bank 2002). However, women continue to earn less than men and are mostly found in sales- and service-related occupations (United Nations 2010).

Although two-thirds of students in tertiary education are female (UNESCO 2003/4) and women comprise more than 80% of the medicine and law graduates from the universities, women are not yet common in the corridors and board rooms of economic or political power with less access to opportunities and rewards commensurate with their educational attainment (UNESCO 1996). Despite this general trend, there have been several female Caribbean Prime Ministers, including the two current Prime Ministers in Jamaica and in Trinidad and Tobago. While the role of mothering and caregiving is a pertinent women's issue in regard to health, there is also an increasing interest in men's roles and notions of masculinity that impact on risky behaviours and an inadequate health-seeking behaviour in the region and elsewhere (Gough and Robertson 2009).

The common experience of slavery damaged family structure, which remains to the present. For example the 2001 Jamaica census data are that among women 16 years and above, 71% of these women were mothers but 59% were single, 17% were in common-law-unions and only 24% are in married unions. Among single women, 61% were mothers (CARICOM 2009). These gender retentions may negatively influence male health, where more permissive parenting of sons, particularly in female-headed households, could facilitate later risk-taking behaviour in these boys. It has been suggested, for example, that this could be related to alcoholism in men (Quinlan 2006).

Box 1. Four main country groupings in the Caribbean.

Four main groupings in the Caribbean

- 19/20 nation English-speaking CARICOM grouping,
- Haiti (full member of CARICOM)
- Small island states, still colonies or departments of colonial powers,
- 3 large Spanish speaking countries with varied political systems, but a shared Hispanic culture

NCD policy responses

Based on the considerations discussed in the previous section it is possible to define four broad regional groupings, based on shared historic and political-economic experiences (Box 1). Although broad, we believe that these groupings enable a meaningful consideration of the relationship between macro-elements of culture and the policy response to NCDs.

CARICOM: the English-speaking countries, a 'culture' of cooperation

A key determinant of identity in the region in present times is language – and the English-speaking countries' political grouping Caribbean Community (CARICOM) was established in 1973 to promote regional integration and cooperation, to coordinate policy and planning, and to develop a single market and economy. There are currently 15 full members, comprising all the independent English-speaking countries in the Caribbean region plus Suriname (Dutch) and Haiti (French), 5 associate members and 8 observers (see Table 1) (CARICOM n.d.).

For historic reasons, Guyana and Suriname, both in South America, and Belize in Central America are also considered part of the Caribbean, and members of CARICOM (Figure 1).

Their shared history, geographic proximity and affinity and the personalised politics of small nation states facilitate regional policy efforts and political cooperation (CARICOM 2007a). This manifests as a long history of successful cooperation in public health issues, supported by the development of regional public health bodies, such as the Caribbean Epidemiology Centre (CAREC), the Caribbean Food and Nutrition Institute (CFNI), the emergent Caribbean Public Health Agency (CARPHA) and more broadly by the Pan American Health Organisation (PAHO). Successes include the early eradication of poliomyelitis, measles and rubella (Irons et al. 1999).

All this forms the background to the historic 2007 watershed within the Caribbean, when the Heads of Government of the CARICOM convened for the first ever NCD Summit by Heads of Government, and issued their 15-point NCD Summit Declaration 'Uniting to Stop the Epidemic of Chronic NCDs', mandating policy initiatives aimed at reducing the burden of NCDs (CARICOM 2007a). The CARICOM has led the way in developing policy responses aimed at the prevention and control of NCDs and was the leading advocate for a UN high-level meeting on NCDs in September 2011 (Box 2) (Kirton et al. 2011, Samuels and Hospedales 2011).

Box 2. Chronology of CARICOM NCD policy initiatives.

CARICOM NCD Policies

2001:   Heads of Government Nassau Declaration "The health of the region is the wealth of the region"

1995–2003, 2005–2009, 2010–2015:   *Caribbean Cooperation in Health 1, 11 & 111 (CCH)* initiative coordinates health policy in the region and is approved by Ministers of Health. NCDs is identified as a priority area

2005:   *Caribbean Commission on Health & Development report* commissioned by the Heads of Government, Caribbean Commission on Health and Development to 'propel health to the center of development' was led by Sir George Alleyne. It named NCDs a super-priority and outlined policy recommendations
2007:   NCD Summit Declaration 'Uniting to Stop the Epidemic of Chronic NCDs' issued by CARICOM Heads of Government at the world's first Heads of Government meeting on NCDs

2007–2011:   CARICOM leads global campaign for a United Nations High Level Meeting on NCDs, convened in New York in September 2011

2011:   *Strategic Plan of Action for the Prevention and Control of Chronic Non-Communicable Diseases (NCDs) for Countries of the Caribbean Community, 2011–2015* tabled at Ministers of Health Caucus, Georgetown Guyana in April

2011:   *Chronic Care Policy & Model of Care for the Caribbean Community (CARICOM) and Framework for Review of Primary Health Care Policy in the Caribbean Community (CARICOM)* tabled at Ministers of Health Caucus, at PAHO, Washington, DC in September

---

About 14 of the 15 mandates of the NCD Summit Declaration address the need for multi-sectorial interventions to address the multifactorial causes of NCDs (CARICOM 2007a). At the regional level, the private sector, through the Caribbean Association of Industry and Commerce (CAIC), and civil society, through the Healthy Caribbean Coalition (www.healthycaribbean.org), are being encouraged to partner with government and its agencies to tackle the risk factors for NCDs.

While there have been significant achievements, in implementing the Port of Spain Declaration on NCD prevention and control in the region, much more needs to be done (Hospedales *et al.* 2011).

Small colonial states

The NCD policies pursued by these small countries are mostly a reflection of their colonial relations and their socio-economic status. In policy area related to external conventions, for example, ratification of the FCTC, they must fall under the laws of the colonial power and cannot act on their own. The five UK Overseas Territories are

Associate Members of CARICOM and their internal policies and programmes are aligned with that regional grouping as well.

The special case of Haiti

There has been a 200 year history of independence, dictatorship and political instability in the poorest country in the hemisphere, where 4% of the 10 million population controls 66% of the wealth, and 77% live on < US$2/day. Recent attempts to return to democracy have been complicated by the destruction of the earthquake of January 2010. Haiti has high rates of NCDs (Figure 2) with diseases of the circulatory system being a leading cause of death. However, communicable diseases have even higher prevalence and mortality rates, exacerbated by the inadvertent reintroduction of cholera by United Nations peacekeepers. It has a weak, underdeveloped public health sector, and there are few NCD policies, no national drug policy, no NCD surveillance, and inadequate systems to deliver services. There is no national exam or certification for health professionals. The culture of dependency continues with reliance on an uncoordinated patchwork of Health NGOs to compensate for an inadequate public system. Traditional medicine is widely utilised by Haitians of all classes (Pan American Health Organization 2007).

Spanish-speaking Caribbean

These are the most populous with a combined population of 25 million, Cuba (11.3 million), The Dominican Republic (9.9 million) and Puerto Rico (3.7 million).

Cuba

Cuba has the only centrally planned economy in the region. The political isolation and the economic embargo created a 'culture' of self-sufficiency and cooperation health care. In keeping with their ideals of collectivism, health care is free and accessible to all through a network of polyclinics, with health teams focused on neighbourhood health education and prevention programmes (Spiegel and Yassi 2004, Cooper et al. 2006). Far from being isolated, however, Cuba has sent health professionals to many Caribbean countries to provide support to their health sector, and has trained many nationals of other Caribbean countries in medicine.

While the health sector is very equitable and efficient, the risk factors for NCDs which lie outside the health sector have not received priority attention. For example, tobacco smoking rates are high (see FCTC section)

Low rates of disposable income, market inefficiencies and the absence of multinational fast food and high sugar drinks, low rates of private motor car ownership are associated with low rates of obesity.

The Dominican Republic

Up until 1978, the Dominican Republic was characterised by political instability and dictatorship. Thus, despite having the largest economy in the Caribbean and an average per capita income of an upper middle-income country, there is great income inequality. The absence of a need to face the electorate resulted in government corruption in favour of the ruling classes and inadequate health policies and programmes for the vast majority of the population. In the 1990s, urban poverty rose from 48% to 66%, while the country health expenditures were maintained at <2% GDP. Only 10% of children, who enter first grade, graduate from high school.

The General Health Act (Law 42-01) and the Social Security Act (Law 87-01) were new laws passed in 2001 in order to regulate public health and health risks, formulate 10-year health plans, and introduce mandatory health insurance, but this has not been fully implemented (Pan American Health Organization 2007).

Puerto Rico

The culture of Puerto Rico is a mixture of Hispanic, USA and Afro-Caribbean, related to their geography and history. Spanish colonialism ended in 1898 when Puerto Rico became a USA possession. They were granted internal self-government in 1952, with later expansion of their role in controlling their own foreign affairs, but the Head of State remains the President of the USA.

Twenty five per cent of the population are University graduates, and the country has a high per capita income. Yet there remains significant income inequality, poverty and high rates of unemployment,

Chronic NCDs account for 8 of the 10 leading causes of death and two-thirds of all deaths.

Aligned with the policies of the USA, in the 1990s, most of the health care infrastructure was privatised and health insurance was contracted out. The profit motive distorted the sector resulting in duplication of services, lack of coordination, lack of psychiatric services and decline in access (Pan American Health Organization 2007).

Framework convention on tobacco Control (FCTC)

The FCTC is the first international treaty of the World Health Organization and the status in the Caribbean is a good reflection of policy adoption influenced by culture, history and current politics and capacity related to population size.

Tobacco policy in CARICOM

All CARICOM countries signed the FCTC in 2003 and 2004, and all, except Haiti, have ratified it, though implementation has been slow. Ratification occurred during 2004–2011, with the countries with larger populations being first to ratify and the smaller countries being tardier. The culture of cooperation in health in the region was a driving force in the ratification by the smaller countries, as the FCTC ratification status was closely monitored by the annual caucus of CARICOM Ministers of Health.

Trinidad and Tobago has comprehensive, robust tobacco legislation which has been shared with the other CARICOM countries, and has served as a model for the development of their own laws. Trinidad and Tobago and Barbados have legislation against smoking in public spaces. Adherence is more complete in Barbados, in keeping with their culture of order, while in Trinidad and Tobago, their inconsistent adherence to the law is in keeping with the more relaxed culture of that country (Franklin Peroune 2011).

CARICOM requires unanimous agreement to implement regional standards in keeping with the culture and philosophy of cooperation. However, this has given an opening to the tobacco industry which has been successful in persuading one small Caribbean country to oppose the implementation of graphic warnings on tobacco packaging. This has stymied the adoption and implementation of a regional standard, since countries now need to implement the standards individually, without the regional standard and support.

Tobacco Policy in Cuba

Although Cuba signed the FCTC in 2004, they have neither ratified it, nor brought it into force. However, there have been efforts to reduce tobacco smoking through public policy, hindered by tobacco being the third largest export, thus vital to the economy. Smoking was banned in public places in 2005, and removed from the ration card in 2010 (Rios 2012). However, these efforts have lagged in comparison with the burden of disease from tobacco.

Puerto Rico, as part of the USA, signed the FCTC in 2004, but has not ratified or entered it into force. However, there are laws which ban smoking in public spaces and prohibit the sale of tobacco to minors, and in 2009, taxes on cigarettes were approximately doubled.

What lessons can be learned from the Caribbean?

This paper aims to review the Caribbean experience of developing and implementing policy for the prevention and control of NCDs and how that has been shaped by aspects of culture. Culture is not only relevant in terms of an acknowledgement of local context – lay understandings of NCDs or political reluctance to tackle cash crop-related risk factors – but can also be understood as a 'policy culture' of regional cooperation. Despite its great diversity, there is a strong history of cooperation on health issues in the Caribbean that is grounded in a sense of shared identity. The example of CARICOM, concerned with broader political, economic and social issues, in addition to health, has been central to region-wide initiatives on NCDs. The 2007 Port of Spain NCD Summit Declaration established a framework for regional cooperation, within which each member state is expected to develop its own policies for the prevention and control of NCDs. This has been facilitated by the development of model plans and policies at regional level, to be adapted and adopted in individual countries.

The Port of Spain Declaration is an example of other high-level regional Caribbean health cooperation such as the control of communicable diseases, most notably HIV/AIDS that take cultural, demographic and social characteristics of the Caribbean into account. It can be argued that ethnic, political and economic diversity is less a hindrance than the grounds for a common Caribbean identity and coordinated policy initiatives, particularly within CARICOM. Other regions might be able to draw from this experience (Alleyne and Samuels 2010). The political and economic cooperative regions in Latin American region, MERCOSUR (Mercado Común del Sur) that link Argentina, Brazil, Paraguay and Uruguay, and the Central

American SICA (Sistema de la Integraction Centroamericano), as well as the Andean Health Organization ORAS (Organismo Andino de Salud/ORAS) could emulate the CARICOM multi-sectorial Port of Spain Declaration.

Aside from regional cooperation, the CARICOM countries have also demonstrated a very dynamic exchange of experiences through sub-regional platforms and openness in embracing solutions that showed success in other countries. Recent examples are the National Health Fund in Jamaica (currently discussed as a model for the Bahamas) and Trinidad and Tobago's decision to provide free access to treatment for hypertension and diabetes through the Chronic Disease Assistance Programme (Bobb et al. 2008).

On a more local level, civil society movements around health are engaged in mobilising different stakeholders, ranging from faith-based organisations to patient groups, to address health promotion with culturally tailored messages and activities. Cultural gatherings such as carnival are used to promote physically active lifestyles in dancing and have informed CARICOM-wide 'Caribbean Wellness Day', and ongoing local wellness programmes.

However, much is still to be learnt. A particularly pertinent issue within the Caribbean is the complex issue of trade and health, and agriculture and health. This includes not only the production of food and alcohol but also issues of import, export and regulatory mechanisms, including the pricing, advertising and labelling of tobacco, alcohol and food products. Policy initiatives here have been slow, and further analysis of the underlying political, economic and cultural mechanisms for this slow response is required. These might include the need for complex coordinating mechanisms that the region has not yet put in place, and consideration of sociocultural factors that can affect the success of implementing policy.

Bismarck is famously supposed to have said that neither the making of sausages nor the making of policy should be watched, both are messy processes (Brehaut and Juzwishin 2005, p. 1). It is clear that in NCD prevention policy measures have a key role, arguably the major role, to play, and the public health community needs to become more involved in promoting healthy public policy. Brownson et al. (2009) have described three domains in which evidence is needed to help guide policy: the content (evidence for what works); process (for example, evidence for how to best implement policy given local circumstances, and what is feasible) and outcomes (evidence on the potential and actual impact of policy).

In work designed to inform policy on NCDs in another middle-income setting, a simple framework (a policy effectiveness feasibility loop, Figure 4) essentially incorporates these three domains and highlights the type of evidence required (Unwin et al. 2010). Within the context of the Caribbean we found few publications describing work that fits within the 'situation analysis', a key part of which is understanding relevant sociocultural factors and which is designed to help guide the process of policy formulation and implementation through better understanding of local opportunities and barriers. As an example of the need for this type of work, there is clear evidence that the perceived importance and relevance of an issue to the public is an important determinant of policy formulation and it successful implementation (Burstein 2003). It is highly likely that successful policy in areas that affect behaviours, such as physical activity and diet, needs to be designed and implemented taking into account current beliefs and practices, and be acceptable to a high proportion of the population it will affect. This raises the issue that the design

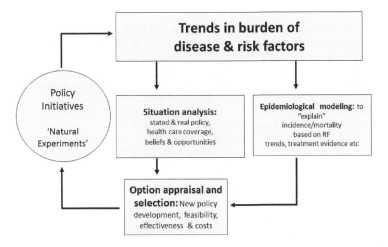

Figure 4. A policy 'Effectiveness-Feasibility Loop'.

and strategies of implementation may need to differ between different cultural groups within the same country.

In summary, we have explored in this paper some of the relationships between culture and policy responses to the large and growing NCD burden in the highly diverse Caribbean region. We have illustrated how broad national characteristics, shaped by shared experiences, can be related to the policy initiatives taken. We have only scratched the surface of an area that is of potentially huge importance to effectively addressing the epidemic of NCDs, and it is clear that further work in this area is essential. Within the Caribbean, for example, work is needed to inform the content and the process of implementation of policies around tobacco, alcohol, physical activity and diet that explicitly considers current beliefs and practices as well as the centrality of tobacco and sugar to many economic livelihoods (Ortiz 1995). There is a lack of evidence for low- and middle-income countries in general to guide policy measures that are effective in the prevention of NCDs, particularly around changing diet and physical activity. Further work to better understand the relationship between culture and policy, and thus inform the content and implementation of more effective policy measures, is needed.

Key messages

(1) The Caribbean countries as an economically, politically and culturally diverse region are increasingly facing the burden of NCDs.
(2) The Caribbean region is leading the effort in the developing world to develop policy responses aimed at the prevention and control of NCDs.
(3) Culture influences policy efforts both in regard to acknowledging local needs and to facilitate regional cooperation.
(4) There is a pressing need for further work to understand what policy initiatives work or do not; understanding the interactions between culture, policy formulation and success will be central to this.

References

Alleyne, G. and Samuels, T.A., 2010. Creating global policy for prevention and control of noncommunicable diseases. *Resources for the Future: Weekly Policy Commentary* [online]. Available from: www.rff.org/Publications/WPC/Pages/Creating-Global-Policy-for-Prevention-and-Control-of-Noncommunicable-Diseases.aspx [Accessed 5 March 2012].

Alwan, A., 2010. *Raising the priority accorded to NCDs in development work at global and national levels – a WHO briefing on NCDs.* New York: United Nations.

Barriteau, E., 2003. *Confronting power, theorizing gender: interdisciplinary perspectives in the Caribbean.* Kingston: The University of the West Indies Press.

Barrow, C., 1996. *Family in the Caribbean: themes and perspectives.* Kingston: Ian Randle.

Beckles, H. and Shepherd, V.A., 2006. *Freedoms won: Caribbean emancipations, ethnicities and nationhood.* Cambridge: Cambridge University Press.

Bobb, A., *et al.*, 2008. The impact of the chronic disease assistance plan (CDAP) on the control of type 2 diabetes in Trinidad. *Diabetes research and clinical practice*, 80 (3), 360–364.

Brehaut, J. and Juzwishin, D., 2005. *The use of research evidence in policy development.* Alberta: Alberta Heritage Foundation for Medical Research.

Brenzel, L., Henry-Lee, A., and Le Frank, E., 2001. *Gender and equity in access to health care in Jamaica and Barbados.* Washington, DC: Sir Arthur Lewis Institute of Social and Economic Studies, University of the West Indies, Mona, Jamaica for Pan American Health Organisation.

Brownson, R.C., Chriqui, J.F., and Stamatakis, K.A., 2009. Understanding evidence-based public health policy. *American Journal of Public Health*, 99 (9), 1576–1583.

Burstein, P., 2003. The impact of public opinion on public policy: a review and an agenda. *Political Research Quarterly*, 56 (1), 29–40.

Burton, R., 2009. Globalisation and cultural identity in Caribbean society: the Jamaican case. *Caribbean Journal of Philosophy*, 1 (1), 1–18.

CAREC, 2010a. *BVI NCD STEPS risk factor survey results.* Port-of-Spain, Trinidad and Tobago: CAREC Caribbean Epidemiology Centre Surveillance Reports.

CAREC, 2010b. *St Kitts NCD STEPS risk factor survey results.* Port-of-Spain, Trinidad and Tobago: CAREC Caribbean Epidemiology Centre Surveillance Reports.

CAREC, 2011. *Dominica NCD STEPS risk factor survey results.* Port-of-Spain, Trinidad and Tobago: CAREC Caribbean Epidemiology Centre Surveillance Reports.

CAREC, in press. *NCD STEPS risk factor survey results.* Port-of-Spain, Trinidad and Tobago: CAREC Caribbean Epidemiology Centre Surveillance Reports.

CARICOM, 2007a. *Declaration of Port-of-Spain: uniting to stop the epidemic of chronic non-communicable diseases.* Georgetown, Guyana: Caribbean Community Secretariat.

CARICOM, 2007b. *Stemming the tide of non-communicable diseases in the Caribbean. Working document for summit of CARICOM heads of government on chronic non-communicable diseases.* Georgetown, Guyana: Caribbean Community Secretariat.

CARICOM, 2009. *National Census Report 2001, Jamaica.* Georgetown, Guyana: CARICOM.

CARICOM, n.d. *The Caribbean Community* [online]. Available from: http://www.caricom.org/jsp/community/community_index.jsp?menu=community [Accessed 2 August 2012].

CDC, n.d. *Global school-based student health survey* [online]. Centre for Disease control and Prevention. Available from: http://www.cdc.gov/gshs/countries/americas/index.htm [Accessed 5 March 2012].

Cooper, R.S., Kennelly, J.F., and Orduñez-Garcia, P., 2006. Health in Cuba. *International Journal of Epidemiology*, 35 (4), 817–824.

Eckersley, R.M., 2007. Culture. *In*: S. Galea, ed. *Macrosocial determinants of population health.* New York: Springer, 193–209.

Franklin Peroune, R., 2011. *Measuring exposure to secondhand tobacco smoke (SHS) in five Caribbean countries: is healthy public policy – smoke free legislation a determining factor?* Unpublished MPH thesis. Faculty of Medical Sciences, Department of Paraclinical Sciences, Public Health and Primary Health Care Unit, University of the West Indies.

Gough, B. and Robertson, S., 2009. *Men, masculinities and health: critical perspectives.* Basingstoke: Palgrave.

Hambleton, I.R., *et al.*, 2009. All-cause mortality after diabetes-related amputation in Barbados. *Diabetes Care*, 32 (2), 306–307.

Hennis, A.J.M., *et al.*, 2004. Explanations for the high risk of diabetes-related amputation in a Caribbean population of Black African Descent and potential for prevention. *Diabetes Care*, 27 (11), 2636–2641.

Henry, F., 2004. The obesity epidemic – a major threat to Caribbean development: the case for public policies. *Caianus*, 37 (1), 2–21.

Hospedales, C.J., *et al.*, 2011. Raising the priority of chronic noncommunicable diseases in the Caribbean. *Revista Panamericana de Salud Pública*, 30, 393–400.

Irons, B., *et al.*, 1999. The immunisation programme in the Caribbean. *Caribb Health*, 2 (3), 9–11.

Kirton, J., Guebert, J., and Samuels, T.A. 2011. *Controlling NCDs through summitry: the CARICOM case study* [online]. Paper comissioned by the Pan Amercian Health Organization/ World Health Organization. Available from: http://www.ghdp.utoronto.ca/pubs/caricom-case-study.pdf [Accessed 4 December 2012].

Miller, G., Maude, G., and Beckles, G., 1996. Incidence of hypertension and non-insulin dependent diabetes mellitus and associated risk factors in a rapidly developing Caribbean community: the St James survey, Trinidad. *Journal of Epidemiology and Community Health*, 50 (5), 497–504.

Montenegro, R.A. and Stephens, C., 2006. Indigenous health in Latin America and the Caribbean. *The Lancet*, 367 (9525), 1859–1869.

Ortiz, F., 1995. *Cuban counterpoint: tobacco and sugar.* Durham, NC: Duke University Press.

PAHO, 2008. *Basic Health Indicators.* Washington, DC: PAHO/WHO.

PAHO, 2012. *Basic Health Indicators in the Americas.* Washington, DC: PAHO/WHO.

Pan American Health Organization, 2007. *Health in the Americas.* Washington, DC: PAHO.

Pan American Health Organization, 2010. *Health information and analysis project: regional core health data initiative.* Washington, DC: PAHO.

Pyne, H., Claeson, M., and Correia, M., 2002. *Gender dimensions of alcohol consumption and alcohol-related problems in Latin America and the Caribbean.* Washington: World Bank.

Quinlan, R., 2006. Gender and risk in a Matrifocal Caribbean Community: a view from behavioral ecology. *American Anthropologist*, 108 (3), 464–470.

Rehm, J., Chisholm, D., Room, R., and Lopez, A.D., 2006. Alcohol. *In*: D.T. Jamison, A.R. Measham, G. Alleyne, *et al.*, eds. *Disease control priorities in developing countries.* New York: Oxford University Press, 887–906.

Rios, A. 2012. *Cubans see their ration cards get thinner and thinner* [online]. Latin American Herald Tribune. Available from: http://www.laht.com/article.asp?ArticleId=364816& CategoryId=14510 [Accessed 2 August 2012].

Samuels, T.A. and Hospedales, C.J., 2011. From Port-of-Spain summit to United Nations High Level Meeting CARICOM and the global non-communicable disease agenda. *West Indian Medical Journal*, 60 (4), 387–391.

Spiegel, J.M. and Yassi, A., 2004. Lessons from the margins of globalization: appreciating the Cuban health paradox. *Journal of Public Health Policy*, 25 (1), 85–110.

The Global Youth Tobacco Survey Collaborative Group, (2002). Tobacco use among youth: a cross country comparison. *Tobacco Control*, 11 (3), 252–270.

UNESCO, 1996. *Report on education in the Caribbean: 1996 meeting of the ministers of education in Latin America and the Caribbean.* Santiago: Regional Bureau for Latin America and the Caribbean UNESCO.

UNESCO, 2003/4. *Gender and education for all: the leap of equality.* EFA Global Monitoring Report. Paris: UNESCO.

United Nations, 2010. *The World's Women 2010: trends and statistics.* New York: UN Department of Economic and Social Affairs.

Unwin, N., *et al.*, 2010. A policy effectiveness-feasibility loop? Promoting the use of evidence to support the development of healthy public policy. *Journal of Epidemiology and Community Health*, 64 (Suppl. 1), A20–A21.

Varona, P., *et al.*, 2009. Smoking-attributable mortality in cuba. *MEDICC Review*, 11 (3), 43–47.

Wilks, R., *et al.*, 2007/8. *Jamaica Health and Lifestyle Survey 2007–8.* University of the West Indies, Mona: Epidemiology Research Unit, Tropical Medicine Research Institute.

World Bank, 2002. *Caribbean economic overview: macroeconomic volatility, household vulnerability, and institutional and policy responses.* Caribbean Group for Cooperation in Economic Development (World Bank). Available from: http://www-wds.worldbank.org/external/default/WDSContentServer/WDSP/IB/2002/09/06/000094946_02082404015643/Rendered/PDF/multi0page.pdf [Accessed 4 December 2012].

World Health Organization, 2008. *2008–2013 action plan for the global strategy of the prevention and control of noncommunicable diseases.* Geneva: WHO.

World Health Organization, 2009. *WHO Report on the global tobacco epidemic: implementing smoke-free environments.* Geneva: WHO.

World Health Organization, 2011. *Prioritized Research Agenda for prevention and control of noncommunicable diseases.* Geneva: WHO.

World Health Organization, 2012. *Global data base on Body Mass Index.* Geneva: WHO.

Index

Accounting for Ethnic and Racial Diversity

The Challenge of Enumeration

Edited by Patrick Simon, and Victor Piché

By the end of the 20th century, the ethnic question had resurfaced in public debate. Every country had been affected by what is commonly known as cultural pluralism, as a result of conflicts interpreted from an ethnic perspective.

This volume explores the ethnic and racial classification in official statistics as a reflection of the representations of population, and as an interpretation of social dynamics through a different lens. Spanning all continents, a wide range of international authors discuss how ethnic and racial classifications are built, their (lack of) accuracy and their contribution to the representation of ethnic and racial diversity of multicultural societies.

This book was originally published as a special issue of *Ethnic and Racial Studies*.

March 2013: 234 x 156: 156pp
Hb: 978-0-415-63113-6
£85 / $145